THE SUM~ I L TWENTY TIMES

BECAUSE SOMETIMES LIGHTNING DOES STRIKE THE SAME SPOT TWICE

FRED RUTMAN

Black Rose Writing | Texas

ISBN: 978-1-68513-156-2
PUBLISHED BY BLACK ROSE WRITING
www.blackrosewriting.com

Printed in the United States of America
Suggested Retail Price (SRP) $21.95

The Summer I Died Twenty Times is printed in Sabon

*As a planet-friendly publisher, Black Rose Writing does its best to eliminate unnecessary waste to reduce paper usage and energy costs, while never compromising the reading experience. As a result, the final word count vs. page count may not meet common expectations.

THE THANK YOU SECTION

Where to start? Later in the book, I mention the guy with the never-ending wedding "I'd like to thank" speech. I don't want to end up with a snoozer like that. As there are literally dozens of people who got me to this point, I've decided mostly to create groups of people that I am very grateful to have in my life.

Dedications – of course, it all starts with family: Hashem, aka God. Then my parents, Al and Cookie, of blessed memory. My bro and Sis, Vinny and Cassie, plus the nieces and nephews who did so much for me. Faux Sis and Faux Bro. Truly, Cassie and Dr. Beatles deserve their own section for what they've done for me. And thanks to Dr. Beatles for the podcast song.

Friends of the book – these are my real-life friends, who are all mentioned in the book. If I miss any of you, let me know and I'll correct it in the next run.

- My work wife Aly
- Hannah Solo
- Gracious
- The Borsalinos
- The Contrarians
- The Spiders
- The Jeans brothers and their families
- Dr. Invisilign and his family
- The Calcuttas
- Mrs. Phelps
- Mrs. Talapia
- Mr. 🔒

And many more. I am truly blessed to be supported by my friends and communities.

The main Med team:
- Dr. Plié
- Dr. Coif
- Dr. Kugal
- Dr. Pedals

The Beta Readers
- Eli Kahuna
- The Calcuttas
- The Vaughan Public Library Writers' Group (and in particular, Daniel Scarcello. (He needs an agent/publisher. Ask to see his manuscript. It's very good).
- The Canada Writes FB Group
- The Delay, Don't Deny Facebook Support Group Moderators (many read various chapters)

And speaking of the Delay, Don't Deny Facebook Support Group Moderators, the founder of the group and reigning Queen of Intermittent Fasting, thank you Gin Stephens. Not only for saving my life (and the lives of many others) but for encouraging me to keep writing, supporting the Dead Man Walking Podcast, and contributing your name and the foreword for this book.

Almost last, a special thanks to Brittney Bitch – You know who you are and what you did.

Last, thanks to Reagan Rothe and the team at Black Rose Writing. Reagan is the mastermind of Black Rose Writing, the publisher who took a never-published repeatedly dead person and took a shot on him. I mean, with my track record, finishing the manuscript wasn't exactly a sure thing.

In memory of those I've lost during this project:
My parents, Al and Cookie, Uncle Sam, Aunties Bev, B, and C, Statler, Marcia, Graphic Goddess, Cake Girl, Mr. Philly 2.0, the latter four all from Cancer.

Simi Abrams – At the age of 24, a young man taken before he had a chance to reach his prime. He loved hockey. If you would like, please consider a donation to the Simi Abrams Hockey Memorial Fund, which provides new and used equipment to youths in need. Simiabramsmemorial@gmail.com

Timothy Epp – January 12, 1971 - July 17, 2022. Tim was a classmate in my MBA program. One of the nicest people and outside the box thinkers I've ever met. Lost to Covid.

Testimonials

The report of my death was an exaggeration – **Mark Twain** (There were a number of variations of this quote, so I picked one. If it's not the exact quote, I'm guessing Mark won't mind).

So was mine. Frikken social media – **Repeatedly Dead Fred**

I have known Fred for 20 years. I have watched his unbelievable medical journey and visited him in the hospital. Throughout all of the crazy things that have happened to him; his battles with health and the healthcare system, his positive attitude and phenomenal sense of humour has kept him alive despite the odds. A must read for those struggling or those looking for an incredible and humorous story. - **Tamar Oziel**

This guy is really starting to piss me off – **The Grim Reaper**

Get in line – **Bill "Digger" Smith**, Canadian Cemetery Association

You have no idea – Jonny "Nails" Pounder – Canadian Guild of Casket Builders

Fred's remarkable wit and sense of humor is sprinkled throughout his unbelievable story, as well as a few F bombs. But when you hear his story, you'll understand why. Along with Fred's story, he shares many valuable insights to self-healing and how he was able to turn his life around through intermittent fasting. He also shares many pearls of wisdom including how to follow your instincts, how to get the medical attention you need, and the importance of having an advocate to speak for you. He also describes how he was able to bring himself to a much healthier lifestyle as well as improve his cognitive function through intermittent fasting, exercise, and mental stimulation with advanced learning. – **Cheryl Ilov**, author of the best seller *Forever Fit and Flexible: Feeling Fabulous at Fifty and Beyond,* and host of the podcast with the best name ever, *The Femininja Podcast*

Some people die at 25 and aren't buried until 75 – **Benjamin Franklin**

Fred died at 48, 52, 57, 59 and 60 and somehow, is still going. We have no clue – **The Wise Doctors of Chelm**

Fred is doing it his way – **Frank Sinatra**

I've known Fred virtually for a couple of years. We met through an intermittent fasting group that we were both moderating in. Fred is an inspiring, funny guy who has been through some crazy experiences that would defeat most of us. While he is funny, he doesn't treat his health as a joke. He has learned a lot and he willingly shares his knowledge with others, building them up in the process. Fred is persistent, resilient and courageous and I can't wait to read his book. – **Annette Cheesman**

Always go to other people's funerals, otherwise they won't come to yours - **Yogi Berra**

I first met Fred when he joined our writing critique group and he shared "The Summer I Died Twenty Times" with us. I was working on my own novel, which also explores religion and spirituality, and so I was really looking forward to reading it. Right off the bat, what struck me about his story was just how funny it was. When you think about everything Fred has gone through, you almost feel guilty for laughing. But that's part of the charm of the book: he wants you to laugh. Sometimes, I would point out a place in the text where I thought he made an error, and Fred would give me what became his classic response: "Sorry, I have brain damage." And he meant it literally. "The Summer I Died Twenty Times" is a funny book that deals with a very heavy subject. As I read, I found myself wondering what beliefs he held that allowed to keep such a positive attitude despite constantly being put through absolute hell. And that's exactly what he explains in the book. I would highly recommend that anyone give this book a read to find out why the man whose heart stopped twenty times is also the Chief Lemonade Maker. If you have lemons, make lemonade. For Fred, the lemons just turned out to be near-death experiences. He has plenty of lemonade to go around. – **Daniel Scarcello, Information Assistant and co-ordinator of the Vaughan Public Library Writers' Club**

Fear of death increases in exact proportion to increase in wealth – **Ernest Hemingway**

If that is true, I have nothing to worry about – **Repeatedly Dead Fred** (Because I've been financially wrecked, it would be a big help if you support my Patreon (crowd funding) account. Being dead really messes with your income).

THE SUMMER
I DIED
TWENTY TIMES

The day was Wednesday, January 23rd, 2019. I was sitting on a stool in my laundry room—slash—office—slash—makeshift podcast studio. That is the day I officially met Fred Rutman, who I interviewed for episode 17 of my podcast, Intermittent Fasting Stories. I was still a baby podcaster, with only 16 prior episodes under my belt, but Fred told me an incredible story I couldn't even have imagined.

I've gone on to record hundreds of other podcast episodes since that day, and yet Fred's story still stands out in my mind.

That story? You're holding it—in even more stunning detail—in your hands.

At the end of our recording session in 2019, Fred shared that miracles only happen in the Bible, but I would respectfully disagree with him.

One estimate is that those with Fred's condition have a less than one percent survival rate when they experience an event outside of a hospital. And, with repeated events, that 1% survival rate gets even smaller. Infinitesimally small. Based on those odds, Fred shouldn't be here with us today. Yet here he is. His whole story reflects one miracle after another, along with a great deal of personal determination and a huge dose of self-advocacy.

Fred's powerful story will inspire you to become your own health and wellness advocate...because miracles may indeed happen, but there is no substitute for becoming educated, asking questions, and standing up for yourself.

Fred's story may also inspire you to look more closely at intermittent fasting as a lifestyle. While his medical conditions are not contagious, his enthusiasm for intermittent fasting absolutely is.

Learn from Fred as you read his inspirational story. No matter what your personal health challenges may be, ask questions and be your own best advocate. And, hey! How about giving intermittent fasting a try? Fred and I both think you'll be glad you did.

– Gin Stephens, *New York Times* bestselling author of *Fast. Feast. Repeat., Delay, Don't Deny, and Clean(ish)*

PROLOGUE

The Summer I Died Twenty Times isn't just a cool or metaphorical title. In the summer of 2009, I was clinically dead twenty times that we know of – heart stopped, no breathing, ready for the toe tag. And then I wasn't. Most times I died, I also collapsed, hit my head violently, and suffered a concussion. Concussions and oxygen deprivation are a pretty terrible combination for sustaining brain functionality. Or staying alive. I experienced memory loss, balance issues, depth perception problems, as well as PTSD and Post-concussion Syndrome, to name just a few issues. It's been pretty awful. It also helps explain why my writing style can sometimes go off the rails on some weird tangents. Real life conversations can be a trip. We know what the medical condition is that caused all this. You'll have to wait a bit to learn what it is. For now, let's look at some numbers and odds.

Roughly 40,000 Canadians and 400,000 Americans die from medical errors yearly. This story is about how I avoided being one of the 40,000. It wasn't easy. Eleven heart procedures in 11 years, being clinically dead dozens of times, concussions, PTSD, brain trauma. defective pacemakers, botched surgeries, cognitive medical bias, learning to self advocate, and digging deeper than I ever imagined I could. They did their best to add me to the total. Many attempts were too damn close. I was told what happened to me was a one in a billion event or series of events. Thankfully, I've beaten the odds every time. I know more surgeries are coming. I'm clearly playing with house money. The question is, will I beat the odds next time?

Of the twenty deaths, the first death was on me - my body malfunctioned, pretty straight forward. All the subsequent times were because of medical misdiagnoses and non-treatment. But come on, we all know dying is obviously pretty permanent. The only guarantees are death and taxes, right? Look at any cemetery. Outside of a horror film, ain't no one coming out of there. So, dying twenty times, one would have to come back to life twenty times. How is this possible? For the conspiracy theorists/flat earthers out there, there was no deal with the devil, witchcraft, Illuminati, or magic bringing me back to life. I don't know about you, but I surely would have struck a deal to simply live longer and better, leaving out the dying parts. To be honest, no one knows what kept bringing me back.

I was told every story needs a "hook" – something or things that give the reader something to latch on to, keeping them engaged. Having written and lived the story, I see hooks all over the place. But that's me. My gift to you is providing some structure, a bit of a treasure map, to ensure you get hooked and enjoy this journey.

Let's turn "one in a billion" into something pretty familiar to most of us: playing the lottery. You don't need to be a mathlete to follow along. Doesn't matter where you play a lottery or which version of lottery, whether you play it regularly or occasionally, or just hear about it. There are stories of people winning big, and stories of many soon losing all their winnings and/or other sorted tales. Regardless, you know the odds aren't in your favour. As the saying goes, the house always wins. Here in Canada, the odds of winning a single lottery 6/49 are about one in 14.5 million. Obviously my one in a billion is significantly rarer. But wait, there's more! (You need to be old enough to recall that tag line from the Ron Popeil late night gadget ads. Or be old enough to remember watching TV and commercials. Or the pre-streaming world, but I digress).

Keep in mind that I am not playing for a financial jackpot. In fact, I had no desire to play at all. Against my will, it forced me into playing for the ultimate stakes - my life. Each time I "played," the odds got worse. Much worse. Let me try to hook you some more. I didn't give any thought to the precision of the one in a billion number. The number didn't really matter to me. Everyone seemed to understand it's a really small number. I had more important things to worry about. Things like recovering from my physical, mental, and emotional battering and getting my life back, so I just accepted that as a valid number. Until someone gave me a reason to challenge that number. And I mean really challenge it.

In April 2022, I was a guest on Dr. Stephan Neff's "Steps to Sobriety" podcast. Stephan is a retired ER Anaesthetist. You know, one of these superstars who has done and seen it all. Fascinating guy who has re-invented himself many times over. You should give his podcast a listen. In our chat, Stephan told me that people who experience my condition outside a hospital setting have a less than one per cent chance of survival. Inside the hospital (depending on the hospital), the survival rate can go up to 30/40%. Certainly not anywhere near the almost 100% save rates you see on TV. Seventeen of my twenty events were outside the hospital. The events in the hospital may as well have been outside, as I wasn't given any treatment and I came back to life on my own. Stephen then added that the odds of survival decrease significantly with each subsequent event. Today (May 11, 2022), I learned that cumulatively, this number gets small. Really small. Indescribably small. How do I know this?

Well, I called our family statistician, Dr. Beatles. What, doesn't every family have a world-class statistician on speed dial? I shared Stephan's numbers with him and asked if one in a billion was small enough. He said no, it's going to be an incomprehensibly small number. Several years ago, a Canadian couple won the lottery twice in seven years. A news outlet asked Dr. Beatles what the odds of that were. He calculated four in ten billion. Off the top of his head, what happened to me is more in the realm of a person winning the same major lottery every week for five years straight kind of odds. I tried doing this on a spreadsheet and it ran out of zeros. In other words, even the mighty Excel couldn't create numbers small enough. Even my neighbour, the actuary, couldn't wrap his head around this number. There really is no reason I should be alive. Or any level of functional.

I mentioned my need to give you structure and hook for the story. In a sentence I never thought I'd write, I'm trying to be your very enticing hooker.

This is a story that checks off most of the foundational aspects of great tales: overcoming adversity, resilience, beating the odds, making a comeback, mystery, humour, sarcasm, cliff-hangers, medical trauma, botched surgeries, medical device failures, and happily ever after ending (it is no longer politically correct to say happy endings).

Even doctors don't believe what happened to me or my level of recovery. The Angel of Death took me off his list. "I've already put in enough effort", he muttered. "I'm done". Or something like that. He's not overly chatty.

Based on the feedback received from sharing my experience on a few dozen podcasts, many find me a source of inspiration and hope. I hope this helps them and their audiences through their own personal trials. I hope this book does the same.

Last, I am writing this as a tribute/testimonial for everyone, be they medical staff, friends, family, people I "know" via social media, or anyone who has come into my world and made me a better person. I wouldn't be here without you.

Even though I've recovered a lot, my brain still is not back to "normal". I apologize in advance, but I tend to think and recall things less linearly these days. Memories and concepts pop up out of nowhere at the strangest times. You know, because of brain damage and all. Like yesterday (May 10, 2022), I have no idea why I had to call Dr. Beatles and discuss the one in a billion occurrence. It just showed up, as do many of the thoughts in the book. And to me, it seemed urgent and needed to be addressed immediately. So, I've made the conscious decision to include many of these tangents as it helps reinforce how one's mind can be altered via Traumatic Brain Injuries (TBIs). These tangents make perfect sense to me, but maybe initially not to you. I'm confident you will catch on. Welcome to the world of non-visible disabilities. My new reality.

I DON'T GET NO RESPECT AT ALL

"When I was born, the doctor looked over to my mom, and apologized. 'I did everything I could, but he pulled through anyhow.'"
–Rodney Dangerfield

If I were to try to sum up my life, the Rodney Dangerfield joke above is a good place to start. Somehow, I just keep pulling through anyhow. I don't know how or why. But I'm grateful I do. P.S. – Most epilogue/introductions are only a few pages. Mine is more of a prequel. It's going to cover a lot of background. I'll try to talk faster so you get to your destination quickly and safely. Emergency exits are at the front and rear of the cabin. So set your reading (or listening if you are audio booking) levels to speed reading or the Advanced setting, buckle up your seatbelts and hang on for the ride.

MY HALL OF FAME DYING
/BRAIN INJURY CAREER
/TIMELINE

Yes, this background is really necessary. It's your roadmap to the story. Planning a trip is sometimes a bit of a grind, so just consider the next few pages as the planning/grinding phase. It will make the rest of the book your trip of a lifetime.

I see my life's timeline in four chunks. My birth (1961, kind of the obvious starting spot) where my untreated brain injury adventure began. I always felt I didn't experience the world like everyone else, but couldn't figure out how to express my concerns or where to look for help. This era lasted until my thirties (1990s) when I found my first medical diagnoses/interventions/therapies via Dr. Narrow, a psychologist. His diagnosis was that I had a stroke either just before or just after I was born. This started era number two, an era of growth, renewed confidence and getting two degrees plus what I consider to be a Master in Adult Education, but I have to call it a Certification. It's a university/departmental turf war – all the same professors/coursework/standards, but because I didn't do it directly through the Faculty of Education, I can't call it a Masters degree. Yes, I'm obviously still pissed about it, although there is nothing that can be done about it. None of these academic achievements could have happened without the brain tune ups facilitated by Dr. Narrow.

Recently (2021), I've learned Dr. Narrow was just scratching the surface diagnostically and therapeutically, because something called neuroplasticity is the current bomb in brain research. Neuroplasticity is a naturally occurring neurological healing process, which we know now can be sped up by "forcing" the brain to gain new skills. Era three came just prior to 9/11, with my relocating to Toronto and reconnecting with Judaism. The intense learning involved with studying Judaism also sped up my neuroplasticity processes. I am now in era four, and what an era it is! May 2009 is when *The Summer I Died Twenty Times* got rolling, putting me in the front row of an adventure like no other – 11 heart procedures, 22 hospitalizations, dozens of concussions, PTSD, Post-concussion Syndrome, and counting. It's now August 2022, in what's hopefully nearing the end of the Covid pandemic (three bouts for me so far). And I'm still in the front row. Oh, and I will jump back and forth in the timeline a fair bit, so be prepared to do a little time travelling with me.

ME? AN AUTHOR?
WHO WOULD HAVE THOUGHT?

There are roughly 40 people in the room. I take a long look around, trying to make eye contact with as many as I can. I inhale deeply, release it slowly. Then I start. "Hi, my name is Fred Rutman. And I've been dead. Dozens of times". Then I take a long pause and scan the room again. The room goes, pardon my pun, deathly silent. This is how I have started off many speeches and presentations over the last 11 years. I have their undivided attention. Because my name is Fred Rutman. And I have truly been dead and concussed. Dozens of times. This is my story. A story of death, faith, resilience, dark humour, cognitive bias, quirks in the medical system, massive communal support, brain trauma, and recovery. Intermittent Fasting (IF) and its healing properties also have to be included/juxtaposed with the havoc that dying has wreaked on my life and career. And of course, what happens when you die. Or more accurately, what happens to me when I die.

I get asked a lot why I feel I need to tell this story. First, this is a story unlike any that I've ever heard. Any time I tell the story to a new doctor, they don't believe it. They don't believe my charts. I often have to get them to call my primary doctors to confirm this is not a ruse of some sort. It needs to be told. My experience is a 100% outlier of outliers of outliers. After all the trauma I've sustained, it's a miracle that I can write a book. Actually, it's a miracle I am alive. Or in any way functional. Here are the stats. I had a stroke at birth, which caused all sorts of brain trauma that no one caught. I have a heart condition called a severe full AV block. Why, they don't know. What they do know is it prevents your heart's electrical signals from telling the atria and ventricle to beat in synch. That is to say, my heart stops. Now I am 100% fully dependent on a pacemaker to keep me alive. Kind of like Iron Man, for you pop culture peeps. I've had four pacemakers in 11 years. Why so many you ask? Because three of the four pacemakers, which rarely break or malfunction, have failed multiple times. Collectively, my heart has stopped 50 plus times. Sometimes for extended periods of time. During many of these stoppages, I collapsed and bashed my head, resulting in concussions/brain damage beyond that of my original stoke, plus Post-concussion Syndrome plus PTSD. The large majority of this should never have happened. To me or to anyone else. But it has. And sadly, it will to others as well. That's just the way the system works.

A lot of this book is being written during the 2020 Covid pandemic. This is a horrible time for many. A few weeks ago (early July 2020), I was having an appropriately socially distanced conversation with my neighbour Ish. Yes, her name is actually Ish. She said that when this pandemic ends, there will be many people lamenting how they didn't take advantage of this imposed downtime to better position themselves for the future. Be it upgrading skills, fitness, relationships, changing or creating a few new habits or routines. I think it was an astute observation. I am in that boat too - although I am always seem to be in some version of self-improvement mode – for a different reason. I am writing this in the midst of an unguided rehab from yet more cardiac surgery. Why unguided you ask? Covid has shut most everything down. I haven't seen a doctor since I was released from the hospital in March 2020 – at this point, it is now August 2022. Usually, one would go through a specific cardiac rehab program, but those have been fully shut down. I have a couple of fitness brochures given to me as I was released from the hospital. Even though I am totally winging it, I'm impressed with the progress I'm making. But could I be doing more?

That being said, I'm trying to do what I've always done – be the Chief Lemonade Officer. I always try to take those lemons – and there have been many – and make lemonade. Check my LinkedIn profile. That's my job title. It's just who I am. Always in some form of self-improvement or growth mode. During Covid, you read so many articles that start off "In these troubling times…". Well, in these troubling times, I am making multiple batches of lemonade. One of them is writing this book. I believe most people have the capacity to learn how to be their own Chief Lemonade Officers at some level. I've seen many stand up to all sorts of adversity. My friend Philly 2.0, for example. You'll read about her later in the book. Each of you will find your own route to this, your own levels, and at the right time. I'm a significantly better lemonade maker now than I was 20 years ago. Experience builds resilience. As I tell many of the Intermittent Fasting people I counsel, feeding your brain is just as important as feeding your belly. Learn, learn, and learn some more. Go to a class. Take on a new skill/challenge. Before you know it, you too will find yourself in the Lemonade business.

I am trying to Lemonaditize (aka recovering) from a combination triple bypass/pacemaker surgery. I was one of the last surgeries done before the hospital mostly shut down non-essential surgeries near the end of March 2020. Rehabbing has definitely been much harder than the pre-surgery marketing material suggested. If you are one of those people who believe all blessings are a curse and all curses are a blessing, I am with you. The "curse" of no formal rehab evolved into the downtime, which allowed all my blessings and curses to align so that I resumed healing and writing. My writing was not exactly going well. Even before this recent medical adventure, I really dropped off the cliff trying to write this book. It was maybe a three-year drop. Because I keep having surgeries that derailed me. I'll talk about how all this started later in the book.

I want to make it clear that I am not a traditional author writing a traditional story, so this book won't be written in a traditional style. In no way will this be considered a long-lost work of Shakespeare or Mark Twain. Or perhaps as I am Canadian, I should say Malcolm Gladwell or Mordecai Richler. Either way, I don't see a Nobel Prize for Literature or a Pulitzer or any type of book award in my future. Maybe, just maybe, a National Jewish Book Award or some other non-mainstream award. But hey, feel free to surprise me with a nomination. Or just share how amazing you think this story is.

There are a few traditional writing conventions I will try to follow. It is customary to start off acknowledging and thanking people who got you to this point. And it is a long list. Although it won't be as long as a groom's speech I recently heard. Oh My God. It was a good 20 minutes of him repeating "I'd like to thank…, I'd like to thank…, I'd like to thank…" He literally thanked everyone he could think of, down to the catering staff who folded the napkins to those who made sure the washrooms had toilet paper. I won't do that. Although I will concede those napkins were folded really well. And despite the alleged Covid panic driven global toilet paper shortage, the washrooms were well supplied. In all seriousness, literally dozens of people played a huge role in getting this book published. And I thank you all.

EVERYONE'S WRITING NEEDS A DEFIBRILLATOR AT SOME POINT

Medical staff often use defibrillators to shock someone back to life. I've come close a few times myself. I needed something, some spark, to get me back on track and writing again. In essence, I needed a writing defibrillator. My spark came from a book I read at the beginning of July 2020. I do not know how I got the book or why I decided to read the book. It was just the next in line of my "to read" pile.

At some point, you'll just need to accept that I go on tangents. It's part of having the "gift" of being a divergent thinker. Albeit a divergent thinker turbo charged by brain trauma. A main tenant of being a divergent thinker means you see creative opportunities/solutions that most people won't. Trying to keep up with my thoughts is very frustrating even for other divergent thinkers. The non-divergent thinkers often don't have a chance – they just hang on for the ride. Layering that gift with various brain injuries often makes it next-level frustration for others. Thus, my tangents. Or as one of the proofreaders of the book said, "The reader needs to be prepared for a lot of change of pace and tone". It's a smart observation.

I recognize that at points this may look like one of those Internet miracle medical cure blogs or vlogs where one is told "If you just keep reading/watching, you'll get to the magic moment you can purchase our unscientifically unproven not really proprietary concoction that will make all your maladies go away while making me, the mysterious owner of this blog/vlog ridiculously rich, so have your credit cards and first-born children ready. And maybe a kidney or liver too." Keep your credit cards in your wallets. All I ask is that you continue to read, nothing more.

The first shout out is to someone I have never met and did not even know existed until her book showed up in my reading pile. It is *Bird by Bird*, by the acclaimed Anne Lamott. As I mentioned, I am not sure how I came into possession of the book. Maybe someone gave it to me during my last hospitalization. It is about the basics of writing a book/becoming an author. I figured I would read the first few pages and see if I liked it. I mean, it's probably a good thing to read books on how to write books if one is trying to write a book. Especially when one is in a severe writing slump. It's written in a very quirky first-person style. I liked it and continued reading. Given the trauma and health issues I've experienced over the last three years, it's no surprise my desire to write fell down the well. Heck, the last 11 years has been hell. From 2015-20, I hadn't written anything substantive for months at a time, going weeks without even trying to write. Anne Lamott and *Bird by Bird* showed up at the perfect time.

I know, I know. The general guidance is if you want to be a writer, open the computer every day and write for at least 15 minutes. Even if it just turns out to be changing a period or a phrase, eventually something will break. My friend told me she knows of a prolific Russian author who claimed if he was blocked, he would start typing his name over and over again, until something broke. A few times, he claimed he wrote his name out 2000+ times until he found something to write. That would be a feat and a half on a computer. But this was back in the day. Note that I said typed. On a typewriter. On paper. Without a word-count! I initially called Bolshevik on this – just the paper costs alone would kill that system. Then I remembered that back in the day, primarily only people of wealth or those who had patrons wrote or produced works of art. So I recant my Bolshevik claim. Speaking of patrons, you can be one of mine by supporting my Dead Man Walking Podcast Patreon account. Hey, if you don't ask...

Not surprisingly, we're off topic. I wasn't even hitting any type of 15 minute a day minimum writing standard. I went from July 2015 to July 2020 without writing almost anything. At all. I know this because every time I save my document, I put the date in the title. Besides my own efforts tanking, I had many professionals say they were interested in contributing their expertise in a variety of ways. Like many (most?) projects, people over promise and under deliver. This has been no different. It does add to taking the wind out of your sails. As of August 24, 2022, almost none of them came through. Yet. Remember though, I am the Chief Lemonade Officer, so I'm working those lemons. Of course, some have legitimate reasons for not helping. Like my lifelong friend, the incredibly talented Graphic Goddess (GG). We met in grade seven. GG offered to do all the cover and illustration work. Sadly, brain cancer took her far too soon. GG, I miss you more than I can express. (P.S. – I spoke to the girls – they are doing well). Others, I guess they have their reasons. Maybe they don't believe in me, or the project. Or both. Or they are legitimately busy. Or just not interested. Or can't face their own demons. Or something else entirely. Doesn't really matter. The right people will show up at the right times to make this work.

Anyhow, I sort of had this delusional idea that if I could just get this book published, it would put me back on the path of resuming my very disrupted life. At least that was my thought process. Except I was missing one small piece — finishing the book. That is, until Anne Lamott and *Bird by Bird* turned my life upside down and right side up. Reading *Bird by Bird* and Anne's guidance to her writing classes (paraphrasing here): Everyone wants to be a published author. But no one wants to be an author. And I was stuck in that exact mindset. I wanted to be the famous published author without having done the hard work of becoming an author. And oddly enough, reading that brief passage resonated so strongly with me that I have been writing six out of seven days since early July 2020. It's now August 2022), so it's been roughly 24 months and counting of solid writing/getting published related effort. Making up for lost time, I guess. I can only imagine what I would learn from one of Anne's live workshops. Now, back to our regularly scheduled programing.

BOY, DO I HAVE A STORY FOR YOU
AKA DEATH BY COGNITIVE BIAS

I know, lots of people think they have a great story. If you have ever been at a social function and find yourself falling asleep on your feet as someone painfully drones on and on, you know most people rarely have that great story. A small minority actually do. I know I do simply because every person I share any part of this story with, well, their mind is 100% blown. Like I said – even doctors don't believe it. I will take a moment to reinforce this idea. I've been dead. Stone cold, clinically, ready for the morgue dead. And not just once. Dozens of times. And then I wasn't. Rinse. Lather. Repeat. None of this wimpy near-death stuff for me. The fully dead option was on the menu and that's what I ordered. The flattest flat line you can get. If I can ever afford a custom car, I want the brake lights to light up like the heart signals on the hospital monitors. The doctors have given me no reason my heart eventually resumed beating. There is an obscure medical concept called The Lazarus Phenomenon, where people come back to life for no apparent reason. You know, as in Lazarus of Bethany, who JC brought back to life four days after his (Lazarus's) death. Last time I looked it up, there were 38 documented instances of it worldwide. But all the recorded instances of it are singular events. As opposed to my dozens of events. Feel free to look it up.

THE EVOLUTION OF THE BOOK TITLE

Who would have thought so much goes into picking a book or the chapter titles? Several chapter names I chose were based on the style used to name episodes of the television series, *The Big Bang Theory*. A combination of geeky, science and fun. I guess I could have called the book The Lazarus Phenomenon. In the TV show Arrow, they have a continuing arc about a life-restoring pool called The Lazarus Pit. Yes, it brought the characters back to life. Along with leaving them with a less than desirable side effect; that effect being a continual need to murder people. Another title choice came via my friend Trophy Wife (her hubby has a business that makes trophies although she claims she would be a Trophy Wife to any man lucky enough to have her). She lovingly calls me *Repeatedly Dead Fred*. I answer the phone to hear, "Hey Repeatedly Dead Fred. How goes? Got a few minutes to talk?" Repeatedly Dead Fred was also her choice for the title of the book. I've decided to use *Repeatedly Dead Fred* as part of my personal branding efforts. After much discussion, *The Summer I Died Twenty Times* seemed to be the most straightforward and obvious title choice.

ZOOM IS NOW A REGULAR PART
OF HOW WE COMMUNICATE

Not that this has anything to do with my story, but I promised Trophy Wife that I would mention her a few times and promote her coaching business. If you have been using Zoom during the pandemic, you've seen some pretty awful haircuts. And a lot of other awful things, including Not Safe for Work (NSFW) shots that you can never unsee. Thanks Hank in Accounting, you perv. In the summer of 2019, Trophy Wife became the proud owner of what she thinks is the most horrific pre-Covid haircut in human history. The day prior to writing this, we were on a Zoom call for a Leadership Course she created (Because, you know, she's a coach). Trophy Wife was complaining to the ten of us about her recent cut and how Trophy Husband was saying all the right things even though she knew he had to be hating on it. Well-done Trophy Husband! Oh yeah, back to my story. And yes, I need a haircut. My last cut was February 2020, just prior to being put into pre-surgery quarantine. It's now April 2021, so 14 months. Spoiler Alert – since we are still in Covid Lockdown number who knows what number, I bit the bullet and self sheered my overgrowth. If Trophy Wife thought her cut was bad…

THE DISCLAIMER

I also want to say this very overtly. This is my recollection/ memories of actual events that happened to me. I hold no one responsible. I may get a little snarky, sarcastic, or dark about describing some scenarios. However, I think most people who have gone through what I've gone through would experience those same or similar responses/feelings. I just had a continuous snowball effect of medical trauma crapinstance (hey, I invented a word!) happen to me. Never mind it being a one in a billion event. Then I had that one in a billion event 4 more times. With odds like these, I should be buying lottery tickets. And winning big. Oh wait, I already buy lottery tickets. Dad always bought tickets, so this is a little connection to him. No wins so far. But I hope that winning a major lottery soon is one of the reasons I am still alive. Note I said one. Obviously, I believe other great things are on the horizon. I also wish I had several dying stories like those "come to the light" people have. I've only had a few out-of-body experiences, which are also very trippy. My stories revolve more around the circumstances surrounding my deaths and the effects on me from dying. Also, some (not all) of those come to the light stories can be pretty suspect. They run the gamut from totally not believable to 100% credible.

In no way do I think this is typical for any of these stories, but *The Boy Who Came Back From Heaven* is definitely an outlier.

It's the 2004 story of six-year-old Alex Malarkey, published in 2010. I mean, even the family name should trigger you that something might not be right. At the time, Alex's story became one of the best-selling near-death books in the Christian publishing world. In my research for this project, I came across bits and pieces of this story, but nothing like the July 2019 Slate article telling the alleged full story. The short version is Alex and his father Kevin were in a traffic accident. Alex was internally decapitated (his spine detached from his brain). Alex survived, was in a coma. Tragically, he was now fully a quadriplegic. Shortly after he emerged from the coma, stories started to float about how he had gone to heaven and his experiences there. The book claimed Alex repeatedly went to heaven and back even after he came out of the coma. Very vivid descriptions. Far beyond what a six-year-old should be able to tell. This turned into a book deal for the family, selling 1 million plus books. *The Boy Who Came Back from Heaven* spent months on the New York Times bestseller list. It spurred a number of other similarly themed books that were also successful. And then everything collapsed. When Alex was 16, he recanted everything to a popular Christian blog and all hell (no pun intended) broke loose. Money went missing, the family broke up, the book was pulled from the shelves. On top of the ongoing traumas to the family (and I hope they get some positive resolution soon), Alex's denial made the Christian publishing world extremely nervous. I say these next sentences very tentatively as I am not a theological expert of any sort. Confidence in what happens when you die is a cornerstone of the belief system. If that goes, it's very problematic. Perhaps this is one reason Judaism is very nebulous about what happens when you die or journey to the "World to Come" (which is what many Orthodox Jews call the Jewish version of Heaven). All this being said, I believe (and this is merely my opinion), Alex experienced some level of what was covered in the book, and others took liberties with what he said.

At the other end of the spectrum, there is the story of the late comedian Sam Kinison, who died in a car wreck. Recently (October 2020), I came across a documentary series on the famous Comedy Store in Los Angeles. I'm a big fan of stand-up comedy. The Comedy Store was perhaps the pre-eminent training ground for many of the great comics of the last 40 years. In maybe episode four, they tell Sam's story, which I hope I do justice. He was an unlikely comedian, both coming from a lineage of Pentecostal Ministers as well as formerly being one himself. He also had some substance abuse issues. I know. Shocking, right? Someone in the entertainment business with substance abuse issues.

Kinison died in a highway accident after being hit head on by a teenage drunk driver. Ironically, Kinison himself was sober that night, a rare occurrence for him. Kinison's friend and long-time opening act Carl LaBove was following Sam's car. LaBove pulled up to the scene, saw Kinison wedged between the front seats of his car, unconscious. Then suddenly Kinison "woke up" and dislodged himself from the wreck. No easy feat considering some reports he still had his seatbelt on. He staggered over to LaBove, then collapsed in his arms. According to LaBove (and others at the scene, including Kinison's brother), Kinison started talking to no one in particular. I think it is safe to assume Sam believed he was talking to someone in Heaven. "I don't want to die. I don't want to die". But then there was a pause, as if Kinison were listening to someone's response. Then he asked, "But why now?" Another pause. He again repeated he didn't want to die. After another pause, he responded, "Okay, Okay, Okay", then died in LaBove's arms. That's a pretty hard story to top. As W. C. Fields's proclaimed, "Never follow kids or animals". I should add - or dying comedians. As unique as that story was, I believe that collectively, my death adventures easily top this or any other story.

WHAT MY AUTOPSY WOULD HAVE SAID

If I hadn't kept coming back to life, my autopsy would likely not have identified the medical condition that has been giving me all this grief. It is almost impossible to catch it outside the period of the actual event. That was a major factor in why it took so long to diagnose what was happening to me. The medical community had zero idea what initiated it. It's normally called a full AV Block (Atrial Ventricular) or 3rd degree AV block. Given how this showed up out of nowhere for me, and about 30 years too early, one doctor labelled it a severe onset full AV Block. The Cleveland Clinic Cardiac website gives a good explanation of the levels of heart block. The medical community also does not know why I came back to life. The Lazarus Phenomenon was never mentioned as an option. This is a story of everything that happened to me, didn't happen, should have happened, might have happened, resilience, relationships gained and lost, how this tore apart my life, and continues to impact me ten plus years later. I also have to tell you what this story isn't.

Again, this isn't a bashing of the medical system. It also isn't me just being a big complainer about everything. Yes, I've had some moments where I haven't shined, but mostly, I've been a beacon of positivity through all this. The large majority of the nursing/support staff loved me. I was just firmly advocating for myself at some points. We all know the medical system is broken, but to tell my story, I have to give you a glimpse of what went on behind the curtain, so to speak. And all my doctors know about this and are ok with it. Some of their bosses, probably not so thrilled. Oh well, their problem, right?

In some ways, this has caused me to undertake additional but alternate paths of self-introspection. Even more than I usually do. Part of the cycle of brain healing is you focus on or think in ways you didn't previously. In other ways, nothing at all. Much of the introspection is only happening now as I develop the book, as it was pretty much impossible to do in the early moments due to the PTSD and brain trauma. There are a few obvious factors for that. Even though I try to be a very thoughtful person and sensitive to others, I am a bit more stoic/detached with my normal emotional state. Some people are like that naturally, some people acquire it through experience or training. I acquired it via trauma as my ability to read non-verbal signals or process emotional cues, which were already degraded from the stroke, took further hits. For example, when the Graphic Goddess died in 2019, I had a bit of initial shock. I knew she was sick, but she hid exactly how sick. When I learned she passed, I was surprised but really felt no loss. As mentioned, we've been friends since grade seven, so I should have been hit hard. Mostly, I felt frustrated that I didn't get to say goodbye. GG had her reasons for shielding me from this, so I'll respect that and not get into a "why would she shut me out?" kind of spiral. As time passed, I became more aware of my not feeling any loss than I was about her sudden loss. I mentioned how weird this was to Dr. Plié, my psychiatrist (She's a former ballerina). She said "It's not so unusual. You are still healing yourself. When your body feels you can grieve, it will let you". And sure enough, that is what happened, although it took almost a year. What else was/is different about my ongoing reflections? Even though my life flashed before my eyes dozens of times, I didn't have the "holy crap!" moment of introspection that people often relate after their episodes. I also haven't had any of those overt "Now that I've survived, I'm going to change A, B, and C about my life" moments.

Talking with Dr. Plié yesterday (June 11, 2019), we concluded my emotional detachment (kind of a catch-all phrase) was likely a combination of my natural self, shock, trauma and not really understanding what was happening to me aka PTSD. Also, as someone who is perpetually working on bettering myself, I likely won't have to go through many of the "I've got to change this or that about me" phases. I don't need to, as I am doing it already. To this day, it is still hard to wrap my head around the fact I was dead. Actually, it's beyond hard. I'm still not wrapping my head around this in any way. How can you? I realize how important sharing my mental/emotional states is to telling this story, so I'll try to dig deep to satisfy your needs.

A LITTLE ABOUT ME AND MY GOALS

Welcome to the "about the author/introduction" section of my story. This book is essentially a buffet or combo platter — equal parts memoir/autobiography/cray-cray story. It is really hard deciding how much of my "flaws" and myself I want to share with the world. It's also part advocacy, part self-help and part humour. In publishing lingo, some may categorize this as a memoir. In the more general category, this fits in the creative or narrative non-fiction genre. The story is 100% true with the author (aka me) having a creative license to tell the story in a more fun, humourous, or interesting multi-faceted way as opposed to just the facts. There are a couple of themes that I'll present now and reinforce later in the story. First, much to my detriment, I have been consistently subjected to cognitive bias/rigidity by the medical and educational fields from birth until the present. Again, this is not to blame or shame anyone. We all have our biases or places we dig in. Second, people seem to be in two camps regarding my experience. They either find my openness about what has happened to me either empowering or find it somewhat terrifying.

In putting this together, I had a couple of challenges beyond actually writing the book. First, my head got battered, so my memory was not remembering as much or as quickly as I wanted. Now, in the summer of 2020, I remember more and more events that are filling in many gaps. It has been like a faucet being opened – the more I heal, the more I remember. The more I remember, oddly, the more I remember. Which is frustrating when you think you have finished a chapter, only to find weeks later that you completely left something out. As you may know, writing a book is hard enough with your full faculties. It is brutal with your memory not cooperating. I also had to weave the story while changing the names and simultaneously describing places, people, and things as non-descriptively as possible to protect the innocent (or me, actually). Describing non-descriptively – now there are two words that normally don't go together. And of course, how many people to share this with in the pre-publishing phase. It's harder than it sounds. Or it was for me.

WHO IS FRED?

Let's get the Who is Fred part started. I am originally from Winnipeg, now living in Toronto. The youngest of three, we are all 3rd generation Canadians. I was told my maternal grandmother was born on the kitchen table in Winnipeg. Then again, my aunt (Dad's sister) used to tell us she was a professional wrestler and could whup our butts if we got out of line, so who knows? OK, she was messing with us, but back then, it seemed plausible. I had a lot of challenges growing up. And I still do. You might wonder why I'm going to take you down this medical history rabbit hole. I believe these events are huge contributors to what led to *The Summer I Died Twenty Times*. My earliest memory is from when I was four or five. I'm told most people have earlier childhood memories, some going back to when they were two years old, but I don't. Actually, I have almost zero childhood memories. There are a couple of reasons I don't, which I will get into later in the book. It is one of the reveals I struggled with sharing. Number one is I didn't want people seeing/judging me as damaged goods or as someone to feel sorry for. Reason number two that I have no memories is from the following experience. My sister Cassie had a neighbour friend over and she was very athletic. We were doing what kids do, just playing. I was chasing Cassie's friend around the house and slipped, splatting forehead first onto the concrete floor. Yes, our house had a concrete floor. The tiles didn't add any cushioning. Mom was in another room and said it made a nasty, horrifying sound. To this day, I still have a lump on my forehead. I was knocked unconscious. Or as the kids say today (NSFW warning), I was "Knocked the fuck out!" Which, we now know means you likely have a good concussion. Off to emergency we went. Well, eventually that is. Mom didn't drive. At that time, there was no real "call 911, have an ambulance show up" system. Interesting factoid: Winnipeg invented a 911 system in 1959. When phones were all rotary dials. And the number was 999. The number that took the longest to dial. Not sure why it wasn't simply 111, but that's a question for another day. Mom called a family friend who didn't want to make the drive and insisted Mom pay him for gas and his time. Never figured out why he was a family "friend". Anyhow, ultimately I got to emergency and waited for hours. Had an x-ray taken, which today we now know shows nothing, so they sent me home with no treatment plan. My first known concussion. That theme would play out many times in my future. Anyhow, back to the challenges.

I WAS TODAY YEARS OLD WHEN I LEARNED...

If you are on social media, you may have seen these memes that say "I was today years old when I learned..."

There are literally thousands of these. Much of what I now know about my challenges is from a position of "I was today years old" when I discovered whatever condition. They happen to me regularly. For example, in 2017, I learned some of my maladies are actually a condition called hemiparesis. Via Wikipedia, "Hemiparesis, or unilateral paresisis, is a weakness of one entire side of the body (hemi means half). Hemiplegia is, in its most severe form, complete paralysis of half of the body. Hemiparesis and hemiplegia can be caused by different medical conditions, including congenital causes, trauma, tumours, or stroke". It's not like the condition isn't well known. I've tried for years to explain to medical professionals that I literally feel I am split in half along my vertical axis, but no one would move on it. We now believe this resulted from the stroke. I'll explain more about this in the chapter called The Brain Trainers.

It wasn't until an article randomly showed up in one of my newsfeeds about a young woman in India who had suffered a trauma and was now hemiparisistic. She described it as feeling split in half, exactly like me. I called up the neurologist for a consult. After a two-hour appointment, he said, "Yep, you have hemiparesis. This should have been caught years ago". My first thought was "Well dipstick, why didn't you catch it years ago? Why did I have to spoon feed this to you to get you on board?" Then I calmed down a bit and remembered I saw him for a distinct set of symptoms resulting from a surgery. Anyhow, we are now looking into what sort of treatment plan might be available to me. Just another day in Resilienceville, the imaginary land where I live. As of August 2022, I still have no treatment plan beyond what I try to create myself.

FRED WOULD DO MUCH BETTER IF HE WOULD ONLY APPLY HIMSELF

I have so many challenges that I used to facetiously joke with my parents that they gave me ALL their best genetics. Both of my parents had near lifelong medical issues of their own to deal with. Pretty sure I wouldn't have coped with their respective challenges as well as they have. That being said, I grew up in the era where, for the most part, people didn't spend a lot of time diagnosing emotional, learning, or physical disabilities that weren't obvious such as cerebral palsy or polio. Any problems I had at school or with social skills were chalked up to just me not applying myself or having a crappy attitude. More than one of my report cards (ok, probably the majority) had the "Fred would do much better if he would only apply himself" type comment. There was never anything about how I might apply myself better. It was really just code for "we think your kid is a dick and we've given up on him". Amazingly, there were never any comments like "Fred could do much better if we weren't such lousy teachers with bad attitudes". Now remember, I know how hard teaching is. After all, I was a college professor. I was also a student. I am not bashing all teachers. Just the select few who made my life a living hell, even though I only realized it was a living hell after I saw it through an adult lens. These are probably the first episodes of cognitive bias/rigidity I experienced. That being the teachers' ongoing narrative that there can't possibly be something wrong with Fred – He is obviously just lazy. In fact, it is just now becoming apparent to me how many challenges I had and still have to overcome. Despite all this, I had a fairly normal, hard-working, middle-class upbringing. Played a lot of hockey and football and rugby, but never made it to any elite level. Although every few games, I'd make a Wayne Gretzky-like pass – you know, over a stick through two pairs of skates, right to my line mate's stick, score! - or score a Gretzky-like goal myself. Well, in my mind anyhow.

It also didn't help that I was an overweight kid (ok, I was fat – those great genes again), a redhead (more of an orange head TBH, or as some like to call it, Gingy) and having way above average verbal skills. My ability to speak and tell stories/give presentations is one of my strengths. Possibly in grade three, I remember trying to learn to write script. My handwriting is still worse than any doctor's and is not getting better anytime soon; However, sometimes I can print fairly well. Those teachers though - literally screaming at me for wasting paper and not trying hard enough. Ah, a kid with special needs, parochial school and teachers trained in the military. A formula for soul crushing if I've ever seen one.

MEET DR. NARROW AND THE BRAIN TRAINERS

It's not easy to write on paper soaked with the spit of drill sergeants – errrr – I mean, teachers. Fun times. I was trying. But if you don't have fine motor skills, you don't have fine motor skills. It wasn't until I was 30ish that I learned why I had significantly degraded fine motor skills. This is reason number one I have so many issues. So how did I find out? My sis Cassie became friends with a PhD student whose hubby (Dr. Narrow) ran a special Psychology clinic for people with learning disabilities. I was obviously smart, but my life was going nowhere. This friend proposed that I might have some brain issues and suggested I get checked out. It sounded ridiculous, so initially I resisted meeting this doctor. For months, actually. But something told me to meet with her hubby. And she was right. I was tested and found to have a severe right brain hemisphere dysfunction. Or in layperson's terms, a good chunk of the right side of my brain wasn't working. Basically, the right side of my brain was working at maybe 50% of where it needed to be. How did they determine this? They have decades of data on the brain and body's functional capabilities to benchmark results against. I'll include a section on this and my adventures in brain training later in the book. Or if you find this kind of thing fascinating, skip to the chapter The Brain Trainers.

Like any worthy goal, I've had to work incredibly hard to overcome my laundry list of brain impairments. Even today

(August 2022) in the middle of the Covid pandemic, I still require ongoing therapy to help me progress. And I continue to learn new things about what other people can do and I can't. This is all just a long-winded humble brag to establish that I am an incredibly determined and resilient person. Kind of a "never say die" type. Or a "never stay dead" type. Remember, I am Repeatedly Dead Fred. Which turns out to be a pretty-good foreshadow of the craziest medical story you will probably ever read. There will also be parts of the story that are kind of dark. As I mentioned, I need to use code names for people and places in the story. So here I am with this amazing story to tell, trying to figure out how to get it published and promoted. I'm going to skip to when, as the cool kids say, the cray-cray starts, with me being a college professor at a business school. Yeah, a professor. No one with half a brain would have predicted this. Oh wait, that's me with half a brain. Who would have thought?

IT'S AMAZING YOU ARE FUNCTIONAL AT ALL

It's early March 2018 and I am sitting with my therapist Dr. Plié discussing my writing this book and other ongoing issues. In early 2010, we started working on the repercussions of my experiences, so it's been roughly eight years of trying to battle back. I started off this session by saying that I didn't know if finally putting this all on paper is simply opening my eyes to a more accurate level of how awful my experience and medical treatment was or if it was just confirming/reinforcing it. Probably both, we decided. Regardless, I was finding it pretty disturbing. About 2/3 of the way through the session, Dr. Plié drops this bomb on me – "After all the damage you sustained, it's amazing you are functional at all". I guess deep down I already knew that, but still. Hearing your most trusted medical professional articulate that was pretty jarring. I actually feel the air and energy get sucked out of the room, but it gives you, the reader, some added perspective. I shouldn't even be alive, never mind attempting to write a book.

A couple of weeks later (late March 2018), I asked Dr. Plié what she remembered from our first sessions in 2010. She had been on an extended leave, and did not know anything had happened to me. I was asking her to help me with the aftermath of an experience that very few other people, if any, have experienced. There wasn't exactly a textbook or template to follow. She pulled out the files and started going through our session notes. Going through my files isn't exactly easy as there are about 10 folders, each about the size of old school phone books (anyone remember those?) to search through. She takes a phenomenal number of handwritten notes. I mean, it's been nine years since my initial trauma. As she leafed through the pages, I tentatively asked her if this would ever go away. "This" being what I now know is called flooding – being completely emotionally overwhelmed. There is no way of knowing, she said. Once again, any remaining energy or air in the room also emptied. Finally, Dr. Plié broke what seemed to be the world's longest silence and added, "I still get emotional about this and it didn't even happen to me!" It's hard describing this type of emotional state that hits me. It's definitely not a pleasant feeling. Dr. Plié said one of her other patients described his type of flooding as a sucker punch. I've also heard it described as a gut punch. I guess with me, it's more like it comes from out of nowhere, just a mass of overwhelmingness, a tsunami of emotion bubbling up from my stomach to my head. I know, I know. Get to the damn story. I'm trying. The background is a vital part.

THE "HI, I'M FRED AND I'VE BEEN DEAD" TALK

A couple of years ago, I was asked to speak to a group of young professionals about building and maintaining their careers and networks. I asked the organizer if she wanted me to cover anything specific and she replied, "This is probably the 10th time we've run this talk. Everyone says the same blah blah. Have you got anything that will put them on the edge of their seats?" I said "Well, I can talk about how dying/being dead can be a real career disruptor". There was a long silence. "Seriously, you know someone this happened to?" I shared the short version of my story and she replied, "That can't really be what happened to you". Anyhow, I gave the talk and started "Hi, I'm Fred and I've been dead". And the 40 people in the room went silent - dead silent (no pun intended – ok, for sure it is intended). Fun fact: Reusing/recycling a previous joke is not only environmentally friendly, but it also reduces my carbon footprint. And then the emotional wave hit me like a tsunami. And the wave freaked the audience out even more than telling them I'd been dead.

Sometimes it makes me gasp, other times it takes me to near sobbing where anyone seeing me can see me transforming and losing the battle to stay in control. That's what happened in this talk. I know staying in control is an illusion because the tsunami just rolls in and, like father time, is undefeated. At its worst, the tsunami takes me to straight to Sobbingville. It may only be for 30 seconds, but it seems like an eternity. It's disruptive, embarrassing, and sucks a ton of energy out of me. And it's equally disturbing to anyone seeing me go through it. Most of the time, it's singular events. Sometimes a double, sometimes a triple. Finally, I asked Dr. Plié what she recalled from my initial telling her of this crazy story. "Shocked" she said. "Just totally shocked. What's even more shocking is that your story never seems to end!" When you can shock a super psychiatrist, you know you've been playing in the big leagues. With that in mind, let's see if I can also shock you.

A PRIMER ON BRAIN DAMAGE, CONCUSSIONS AND PTSD

Brain Damage and PTSD: Of the initial twenty episodes I died, at least 17 of those resulted in my collapsing and cracking my head on pavement, curbs, concrete sinks, or ceramic tile commercial floors. On top of all the other trauma I was experiencing, this resulted in my being concussed numerous times. As an added benefit, I ended up with a world-class case of Post-concussion syndrome. Because, you know, I had to make it as bespoke as possible for me. If you don't know, concussion and Post-concussion syndrome are a hot topic these days. Concussions are a big deal in the NFL and pro sports right now. If you are an NHL fan, you might recall some of the alleged problems Sidney Crosby, Eric Lindros, Paul Kariya and Pat Lafontaine and others had in recovering from their concussions. The Post-concussion syndromes ended the careers of the latter three and continues to affect them to this day. And they all started off much younger and fitter than I, so theoretically their healing should have been easier.

In short, a concussion is a form of brain trauma. Post-concussion syndrome is a resulting set of symptoms that may continue for weeks, months, a year, or years after a concussion. Seeing as it is now August 24, 2022, and this all started in 2009, I am definitely in the years category. Depending on the severity, some practitioners call it a Traumatic Brain Injury (TBI). The symptoms differ for everyone, depending on many factors including what parts of your brain get bonked around, prior injuries, what therapies are undertaken, etc. I've read about everything from light sensitivity (not being able to leave a bedroom and having to keep most lights off) to severe auditory sensitivity, to balance issues, memory etc. It's a pretty extensive list. I lost depth perception, balance, coordination, reflexes, names, memories, and languages. My speech often slurs, among other things. And I did not know if any of this was temporary or permanent. Some of it happened pretty quickly, some of it presented itself much later. Despite a ton of therapy, so many freaking years later, I still have symptoms.

I've since learned about a Doctor in England named Dr. Tamsin Lewis (and this is no endorsement by her, I just came across her amazing story and found it helpful). You can find her story at www.sportiedoc.com/about/. The part I found most helpful was her discussion about brain inflammation and how it just won't show up on traditional tests and scans, yet the patient obviously has a brain that isn't working properly. And if most doctors can't see it on a test of some sort, they tend to conclude that obviously nothing is wrong. I hoped to get her to chat with me and add some more of her experiences, but just couldn't arrange it. I have found that lots of people/experts are excited to talk about participating in a book in the concept stage, but when it comes time to put fingers to keyboard, it doesn't happen. I probably have about 15 people I can put on that list. We probably all could put together a list of people who promised to do whatever and didn't come through. It's just hard to remember that this is often more the norm than the exception.

Besides "the must be seen on a test result to be real" biases, another point I feel needs to be established is every person has built-in biases in how they see the world. I do, you do, police, teachers, old and young. Many of these are unconscious biases, so we don't even know how they affect us. Or those around us. Some biases are very conscious. Or are talked about openly enough that you (or them) have serious deficiencies if you don't know biases X, Y and Z are definitely part of your operating parameters. Racism is an obviously conscious bias, especially when people act on it. Even doctors have it. It got to the point where I felt I needed to ask, "Do you have any proof you are a doctor?" Of course, you can't actually say this out of fear you are going to piss off or insult the person or team you want to help you. Or sometimes you do, like I did recently with an eye doctor who refused to listen to my prior health records regarding my lack of vision in my left eye, which is likely a result of the stroke. Regardless, I wondered about this a lot and soon you will see why.

COGNITIVE BIAS/RIGIDITY 101

At the time this started happening to me, I didn't know what I was experiencing was being clinically dead. It wasn't until about the 16th episode the doctors also clued into what was really going on. Because frankly, they were so caught up in their own medical cognitive rigidity, which can be both conscious or unconscious (Thanks for this concept Dr. Plié). They couldn't get out of their own way to practice quality medicine. Simply put, cognitive rigidity means the inability to transition from thinking about things one way, to thinking about or considering them from a different perspective. They dig in their heels and just become entrenched. You've probably had interactions with people like this. Heck, I've probably dug in my heels a few times myself. Ok, more than a few times, but I am much better at not doing this than I used to be. However, when digging in your heels is your modus operandi, your standard go-to response to everything, you are operating at a serious deficiency. There seems to be a spectrum of cognitive rigidity types. I seemed to experience a continuous flow of medical experts with extreme cognitive rigidity. A great example of cognitive rigidity is the 2020 U.S. election and how much of the country is split into various versions of "Us versus Them" and "Them versus Us" with absolutely no one moving off their position. It can often be painful or humbling to move off your spot. In general, society would be better off if we could all improve this skill and be a bit more humble.

It took weeks and months after figuring out what was going on, to realize the full repercussions of all that dying, oxygen deprivation, and getting my head bashed repeatedly. Amazingly, despite everything that happened to me, I was not given one concussion test, not one visit by a neurologist, not one head x-ray, not one CT scan or an MRI. Zero consideration was given to my brain even though they knew I kept hitting my head repeatedly. Just like when I was in grade school because I spoke well, there could not be an issue. Nor did they consider putting me on a temporary pacemaker. Just another stupid ass decision resulting from their cognitive rigidity.

JUST A QUICK CIRCLE BACK

Many of us have that one friend who things happen to that never happen to anyone else. They meet the weirdest people, have the strangest bosses, or find themselves in situations no one else does. I am that guy. When I tell people I am having a Fred kind of day, they know they are in for a story. Finally, we are back to my tag line "My name is Fred Rutman and do I ever have a story for you". Let the cray-cray begin. This is a story about me dying a number of times, starting in the summer of 2009, what happened to me and some people I crossed paths with. Just to be clear, this isn't the typical "come to the light" scenarios people often describe, like the Sam Kinison or Alex Malarkey stories. It is full out being dead. It would probably help if I simplified what I mean by being dead. Let's start with a common medical definition of dead, which is losing your heart and/or lung function for some significant amount of time. Which describes what happened to me to a "T". And no, I do not know why someone would want something to be described to a "T".

As far as I can tell, when most people talk about their near-death experience, they talk about just that — a singular experience. I wish I could say my experience was singular. I initially died 20 times in 2009, followed by another 20 in 2013, another 10ish in 2018, with a few more in Dec 2019/Jan 2020. Unfortunately, this was due to a system-wide medical clusterfuck.

Again, not blaming, just recalling/describing. Oh, and I recently learned clusterfuck is naval, legal, and medical term, not a swear word. I don't think I can state this often enough; I am not bashing the medical community here – just being pretty direct about the facts. And the facts are the large majority of these/my deaths directly resulted from the medical establishment not being on their toes. They seemed to have decided on what they thought the problem was and were running only tests to confirm their preconceived notions versus diagnosing the actual problem. Kind of like the 2020 U.S. election – let's define a narrative and try to fit a cause to substantiate the narrative. The doctors later told me I had about a 1 in a billion-level event that has totally derailed and changed my life in more ways than I can chronicle. Oh, and then it happened a few more times. Maybe if one of you out there are statistics geeks, you can figure out the new odds.

I quickly noticed the powerful effect my story had when I shared it with people, myself included. Heck, even now telling the story often triggers another flooding or waves of emotion event in me! It turns out that introducing yourself with "Hi, my name is Fred and I've been dead numerous times" is a pretty powerful opener. I had zero intention of trying to write my story until sometime in 2014, when someone suggested that I share the story in a national short story contest. The first prize was enticing, and even though it was 12 days to deadline, I started writing. How hard could it be? I used to be a marketer and wrote all the time. The word limit was 1,800 or so and I blew by that in no time. I sent the entry regulations to my brother, Vinny, the lawyer. Vinny (as in the movie My Cousin Vinny) promptly instructed me not to enter. By entering, one gave the contest owners some ridiculously high percentage of the rights to your story in any form (future novels, screenplays, made for TV movies, movies etc.) worldwide and in perpetuity. I said screw that and kept on writing. If I get enough content, I will figure out how to get it published. Why figure out? Unless you have some sort of celebrity or established social media presence, traditional publishers will rarely take on a first-time writer. The fact you are reading this means I both nailed the content and figured out how to get it published. Plus, besides this being a wild and dark story, there are some life lessons to be learned, especially if you end up in a precarious medical situation like I did. Oh crap, I've gone on a tangent again, haven't I? I promise the cray-cray is coming soon. Just think of these as unintentional cliff hangers. Like for those of you of the right vintage, "Who Shot J.R.?" If you don't know this epic point in TV history (you know, when you couldn't stream anything when you wanted to), this was game changing TV.

Some background about my near-death experiences and me might be helpful. Whenever you see someone on TV or in a movie say, "Trust me" or "Believe me", your automatic reaction is to immediately not trust him or her. I ask you to toss that rule in my case. So first, trust me. This is a 100% true story. Second, I've been told I may be a touch direct, sarcastic (see, direct, a touch) and pretty funny, so my writing style reflects my personality (and for those of you with delicate dispositions, this may or may not contain some fucking swearing). Oh, plus a bit of gory detail. And we can't forget anger – as I write and reflect on this, I am getting angrier and angrier with so many people just fucking up (I warned you about the swearing), my diagnoses and treatment. Third, parts of this story require my providing commentary about certain medical and other issues I experienced, so there will be some abrupt story breaks as I lay things out. Like that isn't obvious already. Fourth, I am not any sort of medical authority or expert, so don't take anything I say as guidance. Go see your appropriate medical practitioner. Fifth, my understanding of near-death experience stories (as opposed to my actual deaths) is that near-death experience stories fall into four general categories:

Just telling the story,

The spiritual story relating to the author's definition of God, heaven or hell,

Can we prove scientifically that God, heaven or hell exist?

The story with how it changed the writer's life.

What makes my story so unique is that I had kind of a Groundhog Day of death experiences (Actual death, not near-death, and The Bill Murray movie type of Groundhog Day, not the Punxsutawney Phil predicting six more weeks of winter type). Plus, all four categories apply to me and I will touch each one as we go. I invite you to come along for the death ride of a lifetime. OMG, finally, the cray-cray. It won't disappoint.

THE BEGINNING OF
REPEATEDLY DEAD FRED: 2009-2013
TEACHING ECONOMICS WILL BE
THE DEATH OF ME

Finally, we made it! My first memory about what I now call Fred's 2009 Summer of Death Tour (I think I might make T-shirts like bands do for concerts) is the first time I died. In reality, I didn't know I had died until many weeks later, after about the 17th of 20 times it happened. At first, I didn't realize how bad it was and didn't take it overly seriously. Later, I clued in and realized something terribly wrong was happening to me. Even when I clued in, there was no "Eureka" moment where all was revealed. As my brain continues to heal, more and more facts are revealed. There I was, marking Economics term papers in my home office. Many people would consider having to take Economics as some sort of a death sentence in itself. Grading some of those term papers often felt like that as well. Next thing I know, I was having the most brilliant fireworks display in my mind, with each explosion throwing multiple competing confusing thoughts and images at me for what seemed like 20 minutes. I actually felt the impacts of each explosion. And when I say felt, I mean felt like some unseen force was battering my body and beating the snot out of me. Upon reflection, fireworks is a much too pretty a description of how awful this was, as I later learned I was truly fighting to come back to life. I had never experienced anything so intense. It wouldn't be the last time, either. I eventually dubbed the beginning of these events as brainquakes. The initial episodes of brainquakes were relatively mild because I was primarily horizontal and stationary. Once I was mobile, it turned the quakes into an entire other level of nasty.

Eventually my eyes opened, and I realized I was slumped over in my chair and breathing really deeply. Totally disoriented. After recovering for a few moments, I thought I was simply extremely tired and had fallen into a weird sleep while grading the papers and had a bizarre dream. I was certainly exhausted at that point. I decided it would be best to call it a night and hit the sack. Unfortunately, the night wasn't over. This was just the beginning of the Summer of Death Tour.

WE NOW RETURN TO OUR REGULARLY SCHEDULED DYING

The simple plan of hitting the sack failed miserably. The next thing I knew, I was experiencing the same fireworks display, my eyes opening to see the pot lights on the ceiling, me flat out on the floor. Finally, gaining some composure (or so I thought), I once again tried to get to my bed. This time I finally opened my eyes while slumped in the door jamb of the bedroom. With some effort, I crawled into bed. As I lay there, I was pouring sweat, feeling even more exhausted and thinking I must have some intense flu or food poisoning – weird but no biggie. People get sick all the time, right? Except it turns out it was a biggie I was so messed up from whatever happened to me that it never crossed my mind that I needed urgent medical intervention.

INTRODUCTION TO THE BRAINQUAKES

Life went back to normal for a couple of weeks. Mostly, I felt my usual self and thought whatever happened to me had passed. It was now Friday afternoon, time to get ready for the Sabbath (Did I mention I am an Orthodox-leaning Jew?) Or as my friend (aka Hannah Solo) likes to call me, an entry level Ba'al T'shuvah – kind of a born-again Jew. This is a bit of an inside joke. It's much more of a joke to me than Hannah. She hates it when I refer to myself as entry level and she never calls me that. But when I refer to myself as entry level (I honestly do still consider myself entry level), she gives me the level and intensity of stink-eye that only a loving Jewish mother can. I often went to Friday evening services (Shabbat aka the Sabbath) and then attended a dinner for youngish professionals at a nearby home. At these dinners, I occasionally played the role of the "Rabbi" and gave a minor light-hearted talk and answered questions about Judaism (which I can do because Hannah is somewhat correct in her view).

Services were running late, so I decided to not keep everyone at the house waiting. To save some time, I cut through the Synagogue's parking lot to an opening in the fence that leads to a pathway. I didn't make it to the fence. It literally felt like I was experiencing an earthquake centred in my brain – thus, my calling it a brainquake. Then I blacked out. Ever see the cartoon where Wile. E. Coyote takes the earthquake pills? If you haven't seen this classic piece of cartoon animation genius, find it online. That's what it felt like. I recall thinking "Oh, this can't be good". Eventually the all too familiar fireworks returned with an added bonus - an enormous lump on the back of my head. I had fallen straight back and seriously cracked my head on a concrete barrier, leaving me more disoriented than previous episodes. Known concussion number one was in the books.

Finally regaining my senses (but not really), my only thought was getting to my friends and not making everyone wait further. Weird, huh? I guess sometimes I think too much about other people's needs. I made it about another 20 yards, the brainquake hit again, my head hit the pavement again (or possibly the rainwater drain/steel sewer-hole cover thing) and I lay unconscious in the parking lot for quite a while until the fireworks returned. Known concussion number two. Yep, they can be cumulative as different parts of the brain get banged around. There were kids playing all around, adults walked by. No one checked on me. Again, having recovered not recovered, my thoughts were to get to the dinner. This time, I made it through the fence opening to the pathway, but just barely. I was sweating profusely, the brainquake returned, then the fireworks and I woke up in the crosswalk. I couldn't find my glasses. I implored people passing by to help me find my glasses, but they just stared at me and walked by. I never found them. Insert your preferred joke about making a spectacle of myself here.

Thankfully, the fog cleared enough (remember how the fog rolled in and out in *One Flew Over the Cuckoo's Nest*?) that I decided to stagger back into the synagogue and get some help. I really couldn't articulate what was happening to me. Now I don't care what culture/team/peer group etc., you affiliate with, if the group is big enough, statistically you are always going to find one or two people who are some combination of incredibly obtuse, socially inappropriate, or just a douchebag. And sometimes you hit the jackpot and get all three. Unfortunately, the first gentleman

I ran into was all three and said to me, "I saw you laying down in the parking lot. What were you doing, taking a nap? That's weird dude". Then he just walked away. How it didn't occur to him that something was seriously wrong, I'll never know. I was dishevelled, dirty, sweating profusely and obviously disoriented and in distress such that I couldn't advocate for myself. I wasn't having any eureka moments to help me out. Eventually, two acquaintances that later became buddies walked me over to the dinner, which I thought was a really menschy thing to do. Especially since it made them late for their own family dinners. I'm not sure why they didn't call a doctor over. It's not like there was a shortage of them in the synagogue (Insert stereotype here). Maybe they tried, and I waved them off. I was just too messed up to recall.

THE FIRST SIGNS OF MEMORY LOSS

Well, so much for me getting to the dinner on time. Most of the dinner was eaten, and I sat sweating profusely for 3 hours. I could not stop drinking water and my clothes were soaked. One guest turned out to be a woman I went to grade school with, in Winnipeg. Her mom was my grade two teacher. Even odder, it turned out she literally lived across the street from me in my mirror cul-de-sac. You know how a cul-de-sac has an open end that runs into a feeder or an intersecting street? Across this intersecting street was another cul-de-sac, essentially our mirror. In five years, we had never crossed paths. As we chatted, she kept asking if I remembered this person or that teacher or some event. And I didn't. I didn't recognize it at the time, but that was the first time I was experiencing some sort of PTSD/post-concussion impairment. A couple of the guests decided I shouldn't walk home by myself and gave me a lift (normally I wouldn't drive on the Sabbath). Maybe someone suggested going to emergency, but I don't recall. At home, I had at least a couple more episodes. Even in my depleted state, with at least five events in seven hours, I recognized I needed medical help. I called a neighbour to take me to the hospital. 911 would have been the better option, but yeah, my cognitive abilities were definitely impaired.

The next day, after a variety of tests, they found I was Type 2 diabetic (my sugars were 23! Normal is 4-6. Multiply by 18 if you want the U.S. equivalents) The doctor who would become my endocrinologist/diabetes doctor was the ER doc on duty, so my sugars were brought under control quickly. I was also totally dehydrated. I guess perpetual sweating does that to you. I might have gone through 4 IVs and yet, didn't have to urinate (I know, TMI). They then concluded that they couldn't conclude anything. They thought I might have had a heart attack, but tests didn't show any of the troponin heart attack enzymes. When you have a heart attack, heart muscle tissue dies and releases enzymes. Besides the troponins, they also test for creatine phosphokinase, both of which they can measure through blood work. My levels for both were normal, so they could tell me what I didn't have, but not what I did have. After about twelve hours, they sent me home with no guidance.

CAN SOMEONE PLEASE
TELL ME WHAT'S WRONG?

A couple more weeks went by with no more brainquakes or fireworks. Then they returned. A couple of trips to emergency, the same questions, the same tests, and the same nebulous results. One cardiologist tried telling me that my prescription sleep aid was slowing my heart and causing all my troubles. Ummmm ok, doc, you saying it is slowing my heart while I'm awake after the drug has left my system? But only sometimes? Yeah, I don't think so. And do you have any proof you are a proper doctor besides your white coat? And get me another doctor, please. Further, somehow the hospital slotted this quack in my records as my family doctor. It took a few years to get him excised. As the fates would have it, this doctor would indirectly have a huge positive impact on my health a few years later. At this point, the doctors sure seemed determined to prove that I was having a continuous stream of heart attacks because no one suggested anything different. All the doctors kept asking the exact same questions. I was fat and didn't exercise enough, so of course I was having heart attacks. Even though probably 20-plus blood tests done over a number of weeks confirmed I wasn't. And it turns out I wasn't. Life went on - the same hits to the head (probably up to 10 concussions at this point), confusion, exhaustion, cognitive medical rigidity, and no answers. If the doctors couldn't even hazard a guess, there was no chance I had any idea what was going on.

The PTSD/Post-concussion Syndrome was sneaking up on me, even though I didn't really know that's what it was. I couldn't believe they had no answers. What's that definition of insanity usually attributed to Einstein? Doing the same thing over and over the same way, yet expecting different results. Einsteins they weren't. Recently my friend Mr. Jeans 2.0 (his brother is Mr. Jeans 1.0) told me a Jewish Folklore story about the "Wise men of Chelm", a fictitious city in Eastern Europe, where everyone was a world-class level of idiot. (Actually, there is a city truly named Chelm, but it is not the Chelm used in this joke. Also, the CH is the clearing phlegm from your throat CH, not the CH as in chair). When you learn of a very questionable decision or idea, the source must be from the Wise Men of fictitious Chelm. That's whom I felt I was dealing with, the Wise Doctors of Chelm. I will get to part two of this joke in a bit.

WHEN MANAGEMENT AND
UNIONS LET IT GET PERSONAL

Soon I had another episode/brainquake and yet another not-so-routine trip to emergency. I knew to keep a "go bag" packed and as soon as I recovered to some degree, I grabbed my bag and struggled outside to meet the ambulance. Except, of course, the trip to get the ambulance to take me to the hospital wasn't routine. None of this was. The city and some unions were in strike mode, including the emergency service providers. Emergency services (police, EMTs, firefighters) weren't allowed to strike fully in the same way other union members were striking – they still had to provide some level of service. Did I mention that this was an incredibly adversarial strike? To the casual observer aka me, both sides (management and union members) let it get very personal. And when that happens, guess what you get? You get a whole other level of cognitive rigidity and disfunction. When the ambulance arrived, they briefly check me out, put me on the gurney and slide me into the ambulance. What happened next blew my already blown mind. The freaking morons left me in the ambulance. Alone!

Because the shift was soon ending, the EMTs and the attending management person got into a huge argument about who was going to the hospital, who would stay with me and who would drive the ambulance back to the station, etc. You know, really important stuff when you are on an emergency call. This is what cognitive rigidity does to you — common sense and your true purpose goes out the window. They 100% forgot about me to the degree that they didn't even set up an IV or get me running on the heart monitors. I remember them screaming at each other, then nothing. Until the awfulness of the post-brainquake fireworks returned. I literally died under their noses while they played petty bullshit adversarial management/union games right outside the ambulance. On the upside, I got to use this as a teaching moment when I was able to return to my Economics students, teaching an improvised management versus union exercise. See, making lemonade out of lemons.

It doesn't get much less professional than that. Ok, it does. At least they returned to see me coming back to life, which is the first time I had a witness to any of this. On route, they had trouble getting my heart rate, yet I was somewhat alert and communicating. Then I was gone again. They saw what was happening and had no clue what was going on. The fireworks returned just as I arrived at the emergency department. At least I was hooked up to the monitors this time. Hopefully, this would give them some clues. See, I'm not just angry. I'm really quite the optimist. Still, this adventure had me thinking I was dealing with the wise EMTs of Chelm. There will be joke number three later on.

Yet again, I went through all the traditional blood work and tests in emergency but this time, they had the bizarro ECG strips that showed me being alive without a heart rate, then not alive, then somehow coming back to life. I asked one doctor if they learned anything from the ECG strip. He said no, either I wasn't hooked up properly or the machine had a glitch. There was no way the strip was accurate. And I'm thinking "But it is accurate. You just can't see it. Think Doc. What if what it is saying if it is accurate? If the fictitious TV doctor House was looking at this strip, where would his brain lead him?" Nonetheless, they finally decided something cardiac related beyond the non-existent heart attacks MIGHT be going on, so they admitted me.

MY ROOMMATE IS A HOLOCAUST SURVIVOR

I told the admitting person I was Jewish and needed Kosher meals. The hospital has a large Jewish clientele, so it is used to this accommodation. It was kind of a relief being admitted. I arrived just in time for one of those delicious hospital dinners. As I settled in, they brought me a nice elderly roommate. I don't recall his name, so I'll call him Mr. Jacobs. He was in his mid-to-late 80s. He was obviously Jewish, and judging by his accent, likely a Holocaust survivor. On the little cul-de-sac I live on, there are 10 homes. Four were survivor families with dozens more scattered in the neighbourhood. I saw the numbers tattooed on his arm that confirmed it. I can't imagine the horrors these people went through. Contrary to what I wrote before, as horrible as I kept feeling coming back to life, I suspect what I went through pales in comparison to someone in the concentration camps.

If you don't know, Kosher is a dietary standard from the Old Testament (Or as I call it, The Testament). Pre-made Commercial Kosher meals are supposed to be served double or triple wrapped in cellophane to keep them protected from potential non-Kosher contaminants. While it's a great system, it makes it almost impossible to open your food with the cheap, crappy plastic knife and fork you get with hospital food. The orderly brings me my meal and I notice it's not wrapped, so I ask what it is. Yummy pork stew, he replied. So I say to Mr. Jacobs, "They made a mistake, it is pork stew. Don't eat it!" Mr. Jacobs pushed the tray away and stated as defiantly as I've ever heard anyone say anything. "Zey couldn't make me eat zis in de (concentration) camps, and zey won't make me eat it here!" Crisis semi-averted. I say semi-averted because now we had no dinner.

This created an entire other issue. They only bring up the exact number of meals they required. They certainly don't bring extra Kosher meals, so there were no meals available for us. Often, the ward keeps emergency food on hand like egg or tuna sandwiches, which we could have eaten. Except the cupboards were bare that day. I asked if I could go to the cafeteria, but was told I wasn't allowed off the floor. It was nearly shift change, so the nurses were off finalizing their notes to update the incoming nurses on each patient. Which meant they weren't available to run to the cafeteria for us. Right on cue, my neighbour showed up with some food. Mrs. Neighbour was home from work sick and heard the EMT screaming match, so she told Mr. Neighbour to check on me on the way home from work. And bless his heart, he had stopped and picked up some food. There was more than enough for both Mr. Jacobs and me. Crisis averted.

THE WORST STORY I'VE EVER HEARD

The next day, Mrs. Jacobs showed up and Mr. Jacobs told her I had saved him from eating non-Kosher food. She immediately took a liking to me. I saw she also had tattoos on her arm. After lunch, they took me for some tests, and I wondered if that reminded the Jacobs of the Nazis taking their friends and families away for "tests". When I returned, we started chatting, and I teasingly asked the Jacobs how long they had been dating. I think she said they met right after the war in a displaced persons' camp. I'm not sure how the conversation switched, but Mrs. Jacobs turned the story into one of the ways she and her little sister survived the war. I must warn you it's a truly disgusting story.

I've heard many holocaust stories, but this one was among the worst. She was maybe 14, her sister was maybe 12. Their parents were taken by the Nazis, probably gassed already. The girls were forced to work in a uniform manufacturing plant, being essentially worked to death. They were barely fed. The younger sister got sick, so Mrs. Jacobs gave her own small amounts of food to help her sister recover. Finally, the little girl was so sick she could no longer work. Amazingly, Mrs. Jacobs found a hiding place in the factory to keep the sister safe. When the guards noticed the sister missing, they beat Mrs. Jacobs, who kept telling them her sister had run away. She was able to continue sneaking her sister food and keep her hidden for some time. Until one day, a guard found the sister. He told Mrs. Jacobs he would keep her secret if he did her "favours". Of course, she agreed, not even understanding what favours meant. This pig raped her a couple of times daily, plus insisted she still meet her manufacturing quota. Then other guards got in on the deal. Miraculously, both she and her sister survived. She never told the little sister what she did to keep her safe. Maybe the bigger miracle was that none of these bastards got her pregnant.

LET'S HEAR IT FOR FRONT-LINE WORKERS

At this point, I have to mention the medical support staff. I know that nurses, orderlies, and cleaners are understaffed, over worked and under paid. And like any industry, you have outstanding performers, poor performers and in between. Most of my exposure was with the nurses, who, mostly seemed at the upper end. At the low end, we have the nurse in Emergency who put in my IV and totally missed the vein, resulting in my hand swelling up to cartoonish proportions. At the high end, I had a truly outstanding nurse code named Nurse 2.0. It turns out she is a second-generation nurse. Thus, the 2.0 designation. My sister worked with her mom when Cassie was just starting her nursing career in Toronto. Always pleasant, knew her stuff, always followed through. A couple of years ago (pre-Covid), I was visiting someone in ICU and guess who his nurse was? Yep, 2.0. Still a boss with a great attitude. Here's a shout out to the support staff and particularly to Nurse 2.0.

Even though there was no evidence I was having heart attacks, they decided to send me for an angiogram. This had to be done at another hospital, so back into the ambulance I went. This was the first time I was fully alert in an ambulance. Let me tell you, these things ain't built for comfort. I've since learned that these inter-hospital ambulances are mostly vehicles the Toronto Ambulance Service got rid of years ago. I don't think shock absorbers are any part of these vehicles. You get seriously battered around, which seems counterintuitive to helping get people to the hospital in the best shape possible. Perhaps bubble-wrapping people before putting them in the WhamBamUlance might be a good idea.

MICHAEL JACKSON DOES MY ANGIOGRAM

It is July 7, 2009, the day of my angiogram. The date might be familiar to you for another reason. The doctor (aka Dr. Angio) who decided I needed an angiogram didn't tell me he wasn't doing the procedure. Not surprisingly, things were running way behind schedule and my procedure was going to be about 1.5 hours or more late. I get wheeled into a waiting room that was basically a large room full of people in ill-fitting hospital gowns on gurneys. Angio comes over to get me to sign a release (really, only 1 in 2500 people die from this procedure. I promise!) while a nurse administers the sedative. As I laid there, I had no choice but to watch TV. And what was on? It was the eagerly anticipated day of pop star Michael Jackson's memorial service. On every freaking TV in the room! His talent is undeniable. I'm just not a huge MJ fan mostly because he just seemed too odd for me, especially being "friends" with kids and chimpanzees. He was definitely a 10/10 on the WeirdoMeter. I've never checked the TV schedule to see if there were any funerals scheduled. So as the doc is talking to me about potentially dying, I have zero desire to watch this freak show funeral while waiting for my first heart procedure.

The angiogram waiting room had at least four televisions set to the MJ memorial. Watching it was upsetting to me, but none of the staff would change the channel. In fact, many of the staff literally stopped working to watch hours of this. I was essentially a prisoner and had no choice but to watch it with riveting tales from people like Magic Johnson relaying how his best memory of MJ was splitting a bucket of KFC with him. Seriously? That was the best? I can only imagine your 5th best story. As my faux Bro said (I have a faux Sis married to faux Bro), this was like running the movie Titanic 24/7 in every area of a cruise ship for the entire cruise. Who wants that? My procedure couldn't come fast enough.

Finally, they wheel me into the AngioLab where the doc informs me that some Resident from Winnipeg will do my procedure. Did I mention I was from Winnipeg originally? Insert your best Winterpeg joke here. Anyhow, she looked terrified, which made me terrified. If you aren't familiar with the procedure, they freeze an area of your groin, then open you up and insert a small probe up the femoral artery all the way into the heart. It's fairly invasive. Today (2020) whenever possible, they do it through the wrist. I've had two more since this one (2018, 2020). They found no evidence of heart attacks or significant blockages (DUH!!!), so off to the recovery ward I am sent. The adventure ends with the doctor giving me a souvenir DVD of the procedure. Which has a minor role to play in an upcoming story. They wheel me to a recovery room with a few other men who also had angiograms. The freezing eventually starts wearing off, and I become acutely aware that I've just been speared in the groin. The nurse basically throws a weighted cold pack at my groin and tells me to put it on my happy place to keep the swelling down. Loving care personified. A couple of hours later, back into the WhamBamUlance and off to my primary hospital, with no new info or possible treatments. So, they sent me home.

DEAD MAN WALKING

Dead Man Walking is an excellent candidate for my podcast title. Be on the lookout for it and give it a listen. As I quickly discovered, walking was a little awkward for a few days as my groin healed from the intrusion. A new summer semester started, and I was back teaching economics, which coincidentally, makes many students feel like dying. (I know I just used this joke. Re-using and recycling a joke is good for the environment. Re-use, repurpose and recycle peeps.) I try to inject real life into my classes. I adapted part of the lesson plan to include a debate of union positions versus management positions. After the students finished, I was able to share my story about the ambulance adventure and how adversarial these strikes can become. Of course, the students were shocked. Finally, class ended, and it was a nice day. Deciding to take advantage of both being able to walk pain free again and the good weather, I started on the long walk to the commuter bus. Generally, it was a 20–25-minute walk. Thinking all was good must have tempted the fates. About two minutes in, the brainquakes started, and I thought, get to the bus shelter. Why I thought that I have no idea. What the hell is a bus shelter going to do for me? Didn't matter because I didn't make it. Crack! Face first onto the pavement. I didn't even make it off campus. I don't know how long it was, but a couple of students happened upon me as the fireworks were subsiding. I was so out of it I didn't even realize they were from my class. Although in my defence, I've always had a terrible time remembering faces. Another bonus gift leftover from my stroke. At this point, all the students knew my medical story. Thankfully, they called 911, then oddly left me there alone. Maybe my class wasn't as good as I thought it was. Or I wasn't as well liked as I thought. Then again, economics – what can I say?

The ambulance took forever to arrive. It got lost because of campus road construction. They refused to take me to the hospital closer to my home. The EMTs were nice and started teasing me about my glasses. Remember the pair no one would help me look for? I hadn't had time to replace them, so I was wearing an old pair with a very dated frame. One of the EMTs joked Elton John needs his glasses back. I had recovered enough to banter with them. They were having trouble getting the IV pole set up and tried to slam it into the holder on the gurney. But it got tangled in the blankets and missed. I screamed, "My leg, my leg! You just speared my leg!" They totally bought it. I smiled, and they realized I was messing with them. That was the second last thing I remember. The last memory was the attending EMT saying, "What the hell, you have no heartbeat. But you are talking and alert". And then I wasn't. Unfortunately, the brainquake hit again, and I woke up to the fireworks in the ER. Which lead to an even Fredder kind of adventure. Remember me mentioning I am a nice Jewish boy? Well, the first thing I saw waking up in the ER is what must have been Osama Bin Laden's twin brother. For most people, I think waking up to that would be truly terrifying. It was to me.

A NEW LEVEL OF COGNITIVE RIGIDITY

It turns out I was right to be terrified. But not because of the Bin Laden part. This "so called doctor" misdiagnosed me (what else is new?) but was very specific about it, claiming I had vasovagal syncopes (pronounced sing-kuh-pee – I have no idea where the G sound in syncope comes from) and there was nothing he could do for me. I would just have to live like this. Via the mayoclinic.org website Vasovagal syncope (vay-zoh-VAY-gul SING-kuh-pee) is when you faint because your body overreacts to certain triggers, such as the sight of blood or extreme emotional distress. The vasovagal syncope trigger causes your heart rate and blood pressure to drop suddenly. It usually first presents in the teenage years, give or take. According to Dr. Syncope, I would have to spend the rest of my life walking around and collapsing at a moment's notice. He was the latest practitioner of cognitive medical rigidity.

I soon learned there were three problems with this diagnosis. One, it is generally not a condition that suddenly presents itself in a 45-year-old, and two, also, I didn't experience the normal triggers like seeing blood or something gruesome like someone breaking a leg. But Dr. Syncope decided what he decided, and he wasn't really invested in looking for other solutions, including dismissing the cardiac tape from the ambulance as being in error.

Oh yeah, the third problem? My heart rate and blood pressure didn't just drop – It turns out my heart stopped completely, my blood pressure went to zero and stayed there. Yep, I was clinically dead.

How do I know all this? Because being fed up with my "care" to this point, I called my cousin, who is an Internist of some repute in Winnipeg. In a 30-second phone call, he told me I wasn't suffering from vasovagal syncopes (see above). He said I likely needed a pacemaker and should be put on a temporary pacemaker right away. I tried to get the resident in charge of the cardiac ward to speak to him. Of course, she refused to. Because what could a doctor from Winnipeg know? We are Toronto, the centre of the universe. We don't need advice from outsiders. And she deemed inserting a temporary pacemaker too dangerous. You know, as opposed to letting my heart stop. Besides, she said, we have paddles right outside your room. You know the paddles they use on TV and in the movies? Someone says "Charging", then they yell "Clear!" and then zap you. Except paddles only give single charges and, as it turns out I would need an ongoing continuous charges. And if temporary pacemakers are too dangerous, exactly why are they approved to be used? It's all so contradictory.

Fun fact # 1 – I eventually got a temporary pacemaker, but you have to wait until later in the book for that bit of insanity. This resident working in the cardiac ward showed a complete lack of understanding of the difference between charge paddles and the need for a pacemaker. Boy, I was winning the jackpot of crap doctors. I wasn't until some point in 2021 that I realized it wasn't just the fact there was all this cognitive rigidity going on, it was that these doctors overlayed it with just being totally dismissive. A powerful and negative combination. Fun fact # 2 – You should read a Wikipedia page on the vagus nerve. It is basically the Internet for all your unconscious body functions. Unfortunately (there's that word again), if something corrupts it, it messes everything up. Not to be too graphic, but if you have ever eaten some food that was slightly off and had to make that mad dash to the washroom, that's your pal the vagus nerve going nuts protecting you. Not to throw shade on the nerve but what happens to vagus doesn't always stay in vagus (sorry, I had to.)

WELCOME TO MY NEIGHBOURHOOD

I had three roommates during my 10-12 day stay. My first one was from one of the Caribbean Islands. When the attendants first wheeled me in, he had four or five visitors, who were praying for him. When they left, he told me they were ladies from his church, but he had no idea who they were. I suspect the church has ongoing outreach programs to aid their congregants. Every synagogue I've been a part of also has these types of committees. Many churches do as well. We chatted briefly after the group left. Then I drifted off to sleep only to be abruptly awakened by a Code Blue for the room across the hall. I said to him, "Too bad your friends left. They would have prayed for this guy too". I don't know if he didn't understand what a Code Blue was, but he responded, "Why would they do that?"

I explained that a Code Blue meant someone was in cardiac distress (which he himself was theoretically in for). He said he was having the same symptoms as I was having and had also been told he was probably just going to have to live with it. I mean, we were in the cardiac ward, so it's the most common code called. He just shrugged his shoulders and kind of signalled "big whoop". I said a quick prayer. Later, the nurses came by and started closing all the room doors. Subsequently, I learned they closed the doors so patients wouldn't see them wheeling out the deceased's body, as he (or she) died shortly after the code blue. Perhaps those ladies from the church praying would have tipped the scales. You never know whose prayer is going to be the one that counts. Anyhow, I guess seeing patients who didn't make it is bad for morale on the ward. Several years ago, I was visiting a friend in a cardiac ward. As I was leaving her room, BOOM! A person from a funeral home was pushing a gurney with a deceased person in a body bag. Him running into me was just bad timing, nothing that was negligent. Regardless, it was quite unnerving, so I can imagine what it would be like for patients already in distress. I don't recall talking to my roomie much after this incident. Except for him commenting when they called a Code Pink. He said that must be a fashion emergency. It's actually an infant in distress.

It was around this time that I started calling friends and family to tell them something was going on. My sister Cassie (the nurse) lives in Halifax and my brother (the lawyer) lives in Edmonton. It was hard calling Mom and Dad as I really had no news for them. They were anxious but could do nothing. They weren't up to travelling here. Just a bad, bad situation. As soon as word got out and despite this hospital being a good 40 km (25 mile) jaunt from my home, people started visiting me, which I very much appreciated. They also started bringing me proper food, as the food in this hospital really levelled up on the horrible meter. Plus, I was getting tired of having to explain to every orderly why I wanted kosher food. I also started accessing my network to see if I could muster some additional medical resources.

SUCK IT UP, BUTTERCUP!

An acquaintance shared that her dad had been a top neurologist but was pretty much retired now. I wasn't getting anywhere with the hospital system, so I begged her to set up a call for me. Which she eventually did, albeit reluctantly. I called him Dr. Drill, because, well, he drills into patients' heads. Dr. Drill did open skull brain surgeries in Canada long before the high-tech drills and lasers came to market. Anyhow, he graciously/quite annoyedly spoke with me and promptly affirmed Doctor Syncope's diagnosis that I was having syncopes and should – I don't recall the exact phrasing, but it was along the lines of just suck it up, Buddy. His advice was that when I felt a syncope coming on, just drop to my knees until it passes. I explained there was no time to do that, but he was pretty dismissive. "Of course there is time," he chided me. Strike one on resource # 1. Another doctor friend is a cardiac specialist who works in a hospital outside the city. He told me that if I needed an MRI, let him know and he would get me set up, which I was grateful for. Apparently there are (or were) much shorter waiting lists in the more rural hospitals. Not sure it would have helped, but I never got a chance at an MRI. This was about the time I called my cousin in Winnipeg.

I THINK THE WARD NEEDS A NEW PURCHASING MANAGER

I guess it was my second day in the hospital, so I wandered the halls out of boredom. I went as far as my cardiac telemetry device allowed, which is pretty much the cardiac ward. And even though I had only been on the ward for a little over a day, I really needed to get out of those new allegedly high-tech beds. They are awful. These beds were essentially rubber air mattresses attached to a regulated compression pump. The pump would constantly inflate and deflate areas of the bed to relieve pressure on your body in the hope of preventing bedsores for those who couldn't move around. Great concept, horrible execution. The pumps were so loud and aggressive that they continually woke the patients.

Plus, the mattresses were made of some sort of rubber, so if one sweated (and we all sweat), it didn't absorb the sweat and you would just lay in little pools of your fluids. There was an easy fix for this (beyond not sweating) – put proper linens on the bed. But nope, we got this coarse, near paper-thin fabric pretending to be sheets that did nothing. Because bedsheet cost control is going to be the factor that balances the hospital budget, right? Yeah, no. As a side effect of my yet to be determined "condition", I tended to sweat a lot, which led me to developing a lovely little case of folliculitis. Never heard of folliculitis? Me either, but it itches like hell. It's when your hair follicles get infected. Large patches of my legs had folliculitis from laying in pools of sweat on my high-tech bed. And if you try to rub or scratch the area to get some relief, you bleed all over, making it even worse. Seriously, who makes these decisions?

Another amazing decision was made by whomever purchased the intercom system in this place. Not only does the bed prevent you from sleeping, but patients are also constantly interrupted by nurses etc., coming to take blood, blood pressure, check sugars etc. I'm no doctor but I seriously question how many lives have been saved or quality of care improved from 4 am blood pressure wake ups. But I digress. Back to the intercoms from hell. I swear they must have scored these from some arena or stadium concert venue overstock clearance. The speakers are right behind the headboard, and they just blast the messages at an un-natural volume. I grew up on Led Zeppelin – I get loud. I often enjoy loud. But this was stupidly loud and hugely disruptive to the patients.

I mentioned my mobile telemetry pack. Basically, it's a limited range ECG that transmits back to the nursing station so you can be monitored. The conduction pads they used were so cheap they had no stickability to them. I guess the glue crop failed and there wasn't enough adhesive available. After a few hours, the pads would fall off and the monitor would stop showing some of my heart signals. And one would think that would trigger some sort of alert at the nursing station, you know, that a patient's heart had stopped or something. Who knows, maybe that's what they wanted. After a number of times spent waiting for hours for a nurse to come in and replace them, I went with a nurse to the supply room to get some new stickies so I could see where they stored them. Then, for most of the rest of my stay, I went to the supply room myself to restore my stickies. You are right. Me having to do that myself was ri-stickulous.

It was either day two or three that Dr. Syncope came by to further ~~creep me out~~ check on me. He said something about wishing he could see the results of my angiogram. Which confused

79

me for two reasons: 1) I thought all our hospitals had access to each other's files, and 2) He had definitively diagnosed me with perpetual vasovagal, so why want to see the angiogram? Fortunately for him, I had my souvenir DVD copy of my angiogram in my go bag (angiogram souvenirs – don't leave home without them!). I offered it to him, and he took it. And that was the last time I saw it. Dr. Syncope came to see me one more time. Naturally, I asked if the angiogram DVD had been any help. He asked what DVD I was talking about. I reminded him he wanted to see my test results, and I gave him the DVD. "Oh, right".

Obviously the schmuck didn't look at anything, so I asked for it back. It was also around this time that I was recognizing my concussions were taking a toll on me cognitively. He replied, "Go ask them at the nursing station". Clearly, he had lost the DVD. There was no reason for the nursing station to have it. If I had been my normal self, I would have told him I gave it to you, your responsibility, go find it. That part of me just wasn't there anymore. There was one more significant clue about the toll the concussions were having on me.

That afternoon, one of my friends brought me my siddur – the Hebrew prayer book. Orthodox Jews ideally pray three times a day. I am only a two-times a day guy for the most part – the afternoon and evening prayers. All my guests had left, and I was set to say my afternoon and evening prayers. I read as much of the service as I can in Hebrew, probably 85%. The less familiar parts I do in English. I open up the book to the afternoon prayer section, and immediately became very confused. I couldn't read anything in Hebrew. None of the letters made any sense. I know maybe half the prayers by heart and still I didn't know how to read Hebrew anymore. I've been reading Hebrew at some level since kindergarten. Even the most fundamental of words, the various names for God, for example, were now mysteries to me. After maybe 15 minutes of struggling to make sense of this, I decided just to do the prayers in English. It's now 2018 and while I can read Hebrew again, I still don't understand much of what I am reading. And I only read at about 70% of the pace I used to read at, which means I have no chance of keeping up with the congregational prayers. I hit my head so hard and so often that I knocked an entire language out of my brain. It also affected my English and speech in general, but I'll deal with those issues more in the PTSD/Post-Concussion section. I am today years old (Sept 2020) when I learned I suffer from Aphasia – just another thing to add to the list. Aphasia is an impairment of language, affecting the production or comprehension of speech and the ability to read or write. Aphasia is always because of injury to the brain - most commonly from a stroke, particularly in older individuals. But brain injuries resulting in aphasia may also arise from head trauma, from brain tumours, or from infections. Great, I got it from both stroke and head trauma.

It was now Friday morning. The staff cardiologist assigned to me also didn't appear overly invested in my case. Monotone, no facial expressions. The only thing remarkable about him was his blandness, so calling him Dr. Bland seems appropriate. At least he decided to try a Holter monitor (a portable ECG machine that continuously records the heart for 48-72 hours) on me for the weekend. Basically, it's a dash cam for your heart's electrical system. It's named for, who else, Dr. Holter. It takes a much more precise deep dive into the heart's electrical system over a longer time frame than the regular telemetry pack does. It's also a fairly old technology (from 1962) and still used recording tapes. In fact, it was the size of the old 8 track cassettes. Look up 8 track cassettes, kids. That was how we used to have portable music. Although it maybe weighs a pound or so, it hangs from a strap behind your neck. Over time, it is quite uncomfortable. In 2019, Holters are now totally digital, much smaller, and less uncomfortable. Back to Dr. Bland.

How uninvested was he? He decided to release me! What is wrong with this picture? We suspect something might be wrong with your heart but have no clue. So go home for three or four days, far away from medical supervision/help, and knock yourself out. I mean literally, go knock yourself out. Crazy, right? My cousin told me not to leave the hospital. That mobile monitor eventually turned out to be the key to figuring out the brainquakes and fireworks. Unfortunately (that word seems to come up a lot, doesn't it?), I didn't need 48-72 hours of tape. I needed less than an hour.

THE BEGINNING OF THE END OF THE BEGINNING

As I was packing up, nature called. TMI? Oh, come on. By now, we have no secrets. My current roomie was a highly entertaining diabetic character that developed sepsis (a body-wide infection) from going on a long charity motorcycle ride against his doctor's orders. He had vibrated an open wound on his butt, didn't get it treated, and it became infected. He was in terrible pain, so he was essentially mainlining Vicodin or some other super painkiller. Based on his colourful stories, I think it's not in my best interests to further identify him.

He was using our washroom, which he did - a lot. It was painful to watch how he had to struggle just to get out of bed. TMI number two. In fact, his washroom activities might have been more explosive than my fireworks. Once before using our washroom, my stomach was upset, so I apologized in advance to his wife, who always seemed to be at his side. She started laughing and said something along the lines of "No need to apologize. There is nothing you can do in there that will come close to what I've been living with for the past 35 years". But I digress. The roommate was doing his thing, so I had to find another washroom. Holter monitor on and activated, I sauntered (always wanted to use that word) to the public washroom down the hall. As soon as I closed the door, bam! Another brainquake hit and I slammed face first on the concrete floor. The fireworks passed. I struggled to my feet and bam, another brainquake. My face slammed onto the edge of the sink counter, breaking my glasses. I ricocheted into the wall before I went completely out. More fireworks. Recovering somewhat, I made it back to my knees, and it happened again. At least this time, I was closer to the floor before I hit my head again. Damn good thing the Holter was still on and running. Eventually I struggled back to the nursing station, broken Elton John glasses, covered in blood, my eye starting to swell, sweating, disoriented. And the duty nurse stupidly asked me, "What happened to you?" What do you think happened? What happened are the same things that landed me in your ward. DUH! Then she matter-of-factly reminded me it was time for me to get discharged. Doesn't look me over, check for a concussion. Zip, nada, nothing.

I went back to my room and refused to leave, having a screaming match with the nurses. Even my roommate and his wife said I was nuts if I left. I won (if you can call common sense prevailing a win) and I stayed over the weekend. Friday evening and Saturday were really slow days. Most of my friends observe the Jewish Sabbath, so I had no visitors until Sunday. To keep from going stir-crazy, I wandered the halls and met some of my fellow patients. I was far and away the youngest person on the ward. I met people waiting for bypasses, valve replacements and one really sad case where the guy had an untreatable virus in a couple of his heart valves. He liked to stand by the window at the end of the hall and just look outside. My friend's brother died from a heart virus issue RIP, M. Anyhow, this gentleman told me he wasn't allowed to leave the hospital, there were no more treatment options, and that he was essentially just waiting to die. How do you end a conversation with someone like this? See you tomorrow? Stay positive? I felt really bad for him. Finally, Monday morning, someone came to collect the Holter. Due to budget cuts, there was no one to read the Holter monitor results until Tuesday. Tuesday afternoon, Dr. Bland, the cardiologist, runs into my room. He breathlessly blurts out, "Holy Shit! Your heart keeps stopping, the electrical is fried and you need a pacemaker ASAP". No shit, Sherlock. Where had I heard that before? This diagnosis was truly such a no-brainer that a few years later, when I reminded my cousin of our conversation, he had zero recollection. He said something like "If it had been a remarkable diagnosis, I'd probably remember. But your case was such a basic read, there was nothing remarkable about it. It's hard to believe it took them so long to catch it".

LET'S HAVE A BLOCK PARTY

Turns out I have a condition where the nerves that carry the signals that tell your heart to beat were deteriorating and shorting out. The technical term is a full Atrial Ventricular block, or full AV block. Some call it third degree heart block. Basically, the nerve network was dying. It means the signals that communicate and direct the Atria to pump in synch with the ventricles were no longer getting through. No signals equals no ventricle pump equals no heart pump. No heart pump, no blood or oxygen to the brain (or anywhere else), lose consciousness almost immediately, then collapse and smack my head violently. I was pretty dead. And then somehow, the signals would get through again and the fireworks returned. Lather, rinse, repeat. In Nov 2018, I was seeing my cardiologist to map a strategy for my future care. I asked if they had any clue why this happened to me. He said for the odd person, something autoimmune might cause it, but for me, they had no clue. Further, if it was an autoimmune issue, it would likely have shown up when I was much younger.

I had several questions for Dr. Bland. I thought I should go back to my regional hospital to be closer to home and help. He told me no, that if I left and went back to my area, they would put me at the back of the line, and I'd likely have more episodes. That sounded reasonable, although it was one of those sounds reasonable in the moment, but something about it seems kind of off. I later figured out what was bothering me about this. If I were going to have further episodes there, wouldn't I have further episodes waiting here as well? And if you knew my heart was going to stop again, and you had something to prevent this happening (aka the "too risky" temporary pacemaker), wouldn't the prudent course of action be to use it? Apparently not. Dr. Bland then told me a nurse or pacemaker technician would be by to give me a tutorial. I wasn't sure why I needed a tutorial. I couldn't possibly have to maintain this thing myself, could I? I don't believe I ever saw Dr. Bland again.

THIS WILL BE THE DAY THAT I DIE

They scheduled me for surgery Thursday July 23rd @ 4 PM, telling me the surgeon was squeezing me in as his last procedure before he goes on vacation. I was definitely not thrilled with this scheduling. There are a couple of givens in life, like never book the last flights of the day because if they cancel, you are screwed. I wasn't thrilled about being under the knife while this guy was daydreaming about umbrella drinks in Jamaica. I also would have thought now that they knew I was actually dying every time the brainquakes showed up, that they would put me in the ICU for better monitoring. Nope, there were paddles outside my room, they said. Did I mention the paddles wouldn't help? Nor would they prevent anything.

At this point, I was now considered at risk of falling (again, no shit), so I was pretty much on bed rest unless in a wheelchair, or on a gurney or with someone (large and very strong) accompanying me. I was sweating more, which should have been a sign to the staff that I was trending downhill. It also was making me a lot more uncomfortable because of the stupid rubber bed system and the folliculitis. Which wasn't treated until I was out of the hospital and saw my family doctor. I was also starting to cramp in my right calf. Like the kind that makes you bolt upright from a deep sleep in the middle of the night. The resident who refused to speak to my cousin dropped in to see me, just as another cramp came on.

This is a rough paraphrase of the conversation. How long has this been going on? A few days, I replied. Jesus Christ, why didn't you tell us? You might have a clot. Even though I still wasn't anywhere close to my usual snarky self, I said, "You don't exactly have a strong record of listening to me". Insert death stare here. That would be her throwing the death stare at me, not me at her. Man, some doctors and their egos. So off she went to schedule an ultrasound to make sure I wasn't experiencing a clot. She (or whomever put the order in) couldn't even get that right.

While waiting for my ultrasound, a nurse who had been trained as a pacemaker technician comes in to give me the pacemaker lesson. She shows me a device about the size of an old pocket watch, the actual pacemaker unit. This particular unit came with two wires which go from the pacemaker, get threaded through a vein right into the heart. One wire (lead) goes to the atria, and one goes to the ventricle. I was told these were more sophisticated computers than those that ran the Gulf War fighter jets or the space shuttles. Batteries last from 5 to 15 years and never need charging. I wish my phone and laptop never needed charging. Pacemakers can come with an amazing array of sensors and programming that interpret when your heart rate needs to speed up (like during exercise) or slow down and beat normally (when you stop exercising). You do exercise, right? She further explained the surgical procedure and some things about how to best recover. I was now an "expert" on pacemakers. I could not envision how much more of an expert I was to become.

As the pacemaker lady left, the lunch people came in with assorted delicacies from the hospital kitchen. Do I need to mention, "add sarcasm here"? For whatever day in a row, they brought something alleged to be fish. I kept telling them I don't do fish and they keep ignoring me. As I waited for the ultrasound test, my friends SWT and Gracious came for a visit. They are amazingly sweet people. Now Gracious, she is just on a higher plane of humanity than most people. She has one of these insane stories about her family being smuggled out of the Middle East. They brought me actual food, as did many other people. In fact, Gracious and others in the community also brought me food while I was recuperating at home. Seeing I hadn't touched my midday feast, SWT asked what was for lunch and I told her some kind of so-called fish. Tilapia, I think. She said she likes Tilapia, so I told her she was more than welcome to my lunch. She raised the heat lid, looked at it, smelled it, squished up her face and said something like "I love fish, but I'm not touching that. It's disgusting". BTW, SWT is a social worker and a travel writer. Check out her blog https://socialworkertravels.blog/ or hire her to write something for you.

If you are in the home of Gracious, there is nothing she won't do for you. At my bedside, she asked permission to say Psalms (prayers) for me. Permission? Only Gracious would ask if it was ok to pray for you. Who would be offended by or refuse this? Of course, in the middle of her praying, an orderly comes to whisk me away for the ultrasound. I felt bad that they made this huge effort and trip to come see me and ten minutes in, the visit gets cut short. I did not know how long the procedure would take, so there was no sense in them sticking around. It ended up taking much longer than it should have. That shouldn't be a surprise at this point.

Of course, the trip to UltrasoundVille wasn't the clean process it could have been. For whatever reason, they built this hospital with a huge horizontal footprint, and it seemed to take forever to get to any testing site. Pretty sure I had to go by gurney, which was almost as uncomfortable as riding in the WhamBamUlance. Why so uncomfortable, you ask? The joints where the various sections of the building connected were far from seamless. Every time we'd hit one, it was like hitting a speed bump or pothole at high speed. Quite jarring. Finally arriving at UltrasoundVille, the attendant hands me my chart and just leaves me in the hallway. No place to register or notify anyone. The technician finally comes out to check my chart, confirms that I am me, and explains what she needs to do. Given the cramps were in my right calf, I thought that must be where the ultrasound would be. It was sort of. It surprised me to learn they had to scan you from the ankle right into your groin. This is where it goes not so swimmingly. The doctor (or whoever) wrote on the ultrasound requisition that the cramps were in my left calf, so that was what she was going to scan. I told her I was the one experiencing the cramps, so I was sure I knew which calf it was.

TURN YOUR HEAD AND COUGH

She complained I was putting her behind schedule. I said imagine how behind schedule you are going to be when they find out you sent me to surgery after scanning the wrong leg. She said the requisition was for the left leg, so she had no choice. Exasperated, I asked if it says you CAN'T also do the right leg? There is no danger to me or any extra cost, right? Fine, she agreed to do both legs. The technician proceeds with the scan. As she gets closer to my groin, she tells me she just has to move "the boys" out of the way to get better access. I wasn't expecting that. Nor was I expecting her hands to be so freaking cold that she didn't have to move the boys – they ran in sheer terror. I'm from Winnipeg and I know cold. Now I know cold on Pluto. Damn, woman. Run your hands under some warm water or something. Thankfully, the boys eventually thawed out and returned home. As an added bonus, there were no clots. But also, no idea why I was cramping.

It was now Wednesday evening, the evening before the surgery. I had a steady stream of visitors, and my room was getting overcrowded. I didn't want to disturb my new roommate, so I asked the nurse if we could all go to the lounge. After all, I was at risk of falling and on bed rest. I think the fact I had about 15 people escorting me helped. Quick tangent – on a recent afternoon, (July 2021), I went to visit some friends nearby, the Calcuttas. A couple we know in common (the Double-Mints) also came and yes, we were all appropriately social distanced. The Double-Mints were part of the lounge entourage. Mrs. Double-Mint asked if I remember her bringing me a set of pajamas that evening. I did. I still have them. Back to the party. We took over the little lounge and had a great time. It really helped to have so many people come out to support me. Having this huge dose of them all at once was amazing. Then the Rabbi called and told me the entire congregation was praying for me and had been doing so every day for the last week. It turned out that the extra bit of being pumped up really helped. Because Thursday morning, all hell broke loose.

BREAKFAST IS NOT THE
MOST IMPORTANT MEAL OF THE DAY

They were bringing breakfast around, which I wasn't even supposed to get because, as many of you already know, they want you on an empty stomach during the surgery. But they brought me breakfast anyhow. Typical. Even though I was on bed rest, I could get up and stretch my legs as long as I stayed connected to the bed. I got up and as I was stretching my legs, I looked out the door and saw a nurse or orderly looking in on me, then boom – brainquake and down I went. When I finally opened my eyes, there were about 15 people surrounding me, about to do, well, I have no idea what they were about to do. Somehow, they got all 280 odd pounds of me back on the bed. 280 pounds of dead weight (see what I did there?) The paddles had been moved beside my bed. The only reason I know that is because they left them there. I don't recall if they had unholstered them or not, but does it even matter? You know how vampires have a lust for blood? The staff here seemed to have a lust to use these paddles on me. Despite now knowing I had a heart block and zapping me wouldn't accomplish anything. Later, I was told my head bounced off the dresser/storage thing at the side of the bed (of course it did), then I took out the rolling tray/desk-type thing. You know you are in bad shape when you don't even notice you have an enormous lump on your head that wasn't there 30 minutes ago.

I need to let you in on a little hospital secret – I had seen/heard a bunch of code blues on the ward. Unlike on TV, the med staff doesn't arrive in 8.3 seconds with everything perfectly coordinated and ready to go. I was definitely dead for a while. But the death tour continued and even THEY (the medical staff) were visibly upset now, finally recognizing that they had been taking my situation way too lightly. Even on bed rest, I managed to crack my head again. I was pretty rattled. Now guess what these medical geniuses from the Chelm Medical University did next? You got it. They left me alone again. No temporary pacemaker. No staff. Just. Alone. Well, that's not completely true. The previous day, they had switched out my roomie for an elderly gentleman whose kid told me had been in Canada for 40 years. He was definitely not an English as a first language person. I mean, he spoke zero English, although his kids did. Like many immigrants, when he arrived in Canada, he found work and all his resources through his ethnic network, so he really did not need to learn English. He didn't understand what was going on and was also totally shook up. Soon he would experience an entirely new level of shook up. And me a new level of rattled.

My bed rest rules were tightened up. Now I could no longer get out of bed to stretch. About an hour later, to quote Yogi Berra, it was déjà vu all over again. I looked to the doorway and again see a nurse or orderly looking in. I think they should have stopped looking in on me because boom again, brainquake. This time when I opened my eyes, there was someone about to hit me with the paddles yelling CLEAR!!! There were so many people in the room that they pulled my roommate out into the hall, bed and all. Judging from how crappy I felt and the reaction of the crowd, I must have been dead quite a bit longer than in previous episodes. This was definitely the worst I had ever felt, even though I didn't hit my head this time. And if they had time to get the roomie out and all those people in, it must have been a while. But even that close call wasn't enough to leave someone with me. About an hour later, someone finally came in to tell me they were moving me to the Cardiac ICU and moving up my surgery. Ya think? I think the Wise Men of Chelm started making jokes about the Wise Medical Staffs of the Greater Toronto Area. Thanks to Mr. Jeans 2.0 and Papa Pop Star (his daughter is a pop star) for that Wise Men of Chelm joke. Look, this is all pretty dark, so sometimes you just have to make or write jokes to make yourself laugh. It's a good coping technique.

I was pretty scrambled by this time, physically, mentally, and emotionally. I need to share some extra insight on how awful the coming back to life is. In the chapter "Yes, I Really Understand Pain" I establish I understand a wide range of awful. Nothing I experienced before this even registers a blip on the coming-back-to-life meter. Imagine being buried alive, finally waking up thousands of feet below the earth's surface, suffocating but somehow realizing your situation, then being slowly dragged by your soul back to the world of the living. All the while feeling pain at indescribable levels. I wish this on no one. The dying part was comparatively easy. The coming back to life part, while I am grateful for it, I believe is as awful an experience as I've ever had. Darn tangents. I guess I should get back to the story. I'm really trying to stay on track. I really am. I blame this on brain trauma. From what I can recall, my hours in ICU were quite uneventful. Then again, by this time, my recall of anything was pretty suspect.

Cassie was supposed to be here for the surgery, but she hadn't arrived yet. She and her hubby (Dr. Beatles) were interrupting their vacation in Montreal to come be with me. Just for Laughs Comedy Festival versus my Clusterfuck Cardiac Festival. Hard choice for her to make, but in the end, they came to help me. I tried calling them, but there was something interrupting cell signals in the ICU. In the interim, my friend "Aly" called on the ICU landline and I freely admit I have zero recollection of this call. If this story ever gets made into a movie, I might suggest Alyson Hannigan play her role, thus the name "Aly". A few years later, she (the pretend Aly, not the real actress) and I filmed a commercial where we played hubby and wife, thus attaining her eternal status as my work wife. I recently (in 2020) asked "Aly" if she remembered anything specific from our call. She said I was lucid, described everything that was going on and when she got off the phone, she was in a state of shock over how insane this situation was. As I said, I have zero recollection of this call.

To my amazement, they decided my case was urgent enough to jump the queue a bit more and move me from the 4 PM slot to 1 PMish. I still couldn't get in touch with Cassie, and it was time to head to surgery. I had many new nurses and I tried asking their names, hoping to keep them straight. It was no use. Between all the masks, my brain being extra scrambled added to my already established difficulties recognizing people, I had no idea who was who. A buddy from synagogue showed up right as they were trying to wheel me out to surgery. While it was great to see him, he wouldn't stop talking, and the nurses weren't doing anything about it. Basically, we were parked in the middle of a hallway. Finally, I said "I really appreciate you coming to visit but I think they want to go save my life, so we need to go". And he continued talking us down the hall until we went through the swinging doors to the operating room. He might still be talking for all I know. Hey, some people are just talkers. What can you do?

I DON'T THINK MY SURGERY
WENT AS PLANNED

I think the anesthetist dropped in on me the day before to talk about something or other. The surgeon, I don't think dropped in. Totally different from on TV shows where the warm compassionate surgical team shows up to explain everything and to ease your fears. Perhaps he (the surgeon) was pissed I might interfere with his vacation. I only remember the surgeon and anesthetist being in the operating room, but based on other subsequent surgeries, there had to have been more staff in there. I mean, there had to be, right? I get slid onto the operating table. Someone positioned the instrument tray right over my face and acted as if I wasn't there. I mean, like two inches over my face. It was unnerving and a touch claustrophobic, and I've never been claustrophobic (enter first signs of PTSD). The surgeon and the anesthetist started talking about something that: either freaked me out, seemed wrong to me or maybe just was interesting to me. I honestly don't recall. What I do recall is asking for someone to move the tray and a couple of other questions and being completely ignored. Evidently, I wasn't part of the cool cardiac kids' club.

Finally, they just gassed me without even saying they were going to do it. No "count back from 100…" At least that is what I used to think. Upon reflection, I didn't have the anaesthesia mask on. I couldn't have had the facemask on for the gas because there was no room with the tray being so close to my face. I also don't recall being set up for an IV injection, nor anyone asking me to count backwards. I was just out. Again, based on subsequent surgeries, I am now wondering if I coded (my heart stopped) on the table before the surgery even began and no one even told me. That might explain how crappy I felt after the surgery, although to be fair, I felt super crappy going in. The surgery was apparently successful. At least no one told me differently. I'm going to order the post-surgery report, even though I know they leave out 90% of what went on. Note: As of Aug 2022, the report still hasn't been digitized and is not available to me. I now had a fully functioning pacemaker implanted. No more dying for me. Unless I do (foreshadowing). It's 2021. This freaking adventure just never ends. Just like that kids' song "This is the song that doesn't end, yes, it goes on and on my friends..." Sing along with me, won't you? You won't believe what's coming.

When I woke up, my sister and bro-in-law (aka Dr. Beatles – a huge Beatles fan and he often uses them in his academic research) had arrived safely, albeit a tad stressed and exhausted. They had a horrible time getting to Toronto from Montreal. I feel I have to blame this on Climate Change/Global Warming. Heck, some might even blame this on Trump. They got caught in the worst thunderstorm they had ever seen. Having grown up in Winnipeg, Cassie and I were used to these epic "once a century" prairie thunderstorms rolling in, a couple of times a summer. In fact, when we were little, our parents didn't want us to be afraid of thunder and lightning, so we often went for family drives during storms. If a storm scared her, it must have been something. There is something about driving on the 401 (aka the major east-west highway in Ontario) that just makes people nuts. Visibility on the 401 was so bad that everyone was just pulling over. If you've ever experienced the 401, even in traffic jams, people try to creep. Even if it's just an inch per hour. But voluntarily pulling over? Unheard of. I remember the first time I drove the 401. I was going on a date, which turned into a date from hell, but that's another story. I was probably doing 115 kph, and this person was right on my bumper. I sped up. So did he (or she or whatever pronoun you want to use). This kept going until I was going close to 140. I took the next exit just to get rid of this nutbar, who likely motored on to harass other drivers. The person is probably high-speed tailgating someone as you read this.

CASSIE THE SUPER NURSE

A little background about my sister. Cassie has had quite the nursing career and worked in many areas in several hospitals, so she really knows her stuff. I sensed she was alarmed at how shitty I looked after the surgery. When I got home the next day, I saw for myself how bad I looked. I must have looked terrible right out of surgery. Something was definitely off. Her Spidey sense was tingling. Previously, I mentioned the fog from *One Flew Over the Cuckoo's Nest*. The chief protagonist in the story was Nurse Ratched. If I remember my Grade 12 English correctly (and that's a big if), "Ratched" is a play on words for wretched. While my overnight nurse in ICU wasn't quite Nurse Ratched, she sure was her "mini me". Oh, who am I kidding? She was full bore Nurse Ratched. Just to clarify, while Cassie is a nurse, she is definitely NOT a Nurse Ratched type.

ENTER NURSE RATCHED

As I recall, Cassie and Dr. Beatles went to check into their hotel and grab some dinner. They returned around shift change, just as the super nice nurse was changing over (insert foreboding movie music here) so Nurse Ratched could take over for the night shift. I had always assumed ICU staffs were like Seal Team Six, best of the best of the best. Maybe she was just having a really off day. Or week. Or decade. Somehow, like the computers in The Terminator movie, she became sentient about my having previously used a CPAP (continuous positive airway pressure) machine. You use a CPAP machine to offset sleep apnea. It basically inflates you to keep your airways open, so you don't stop breathing. I had minor sleep apnea previously and having lost weight (yep, at one point I was 340 pounds), I was "cured". The doctor said I didn't need to use the CPAP anymore.

This wasn't good enough for Nurse Ratched. She was convinced I needed to be re-indoctrinated/educated about CPAPs and why they were so important. She brought me some literature and insisted I read it in front of her. I was in no shape to read and process anything, but Nurse Ratched was like a dog with a bone. She wouldn't let up. If I was in my normal state, I probably would have told her less than diplomatically to get out of my face or I will give you a horrible review on Yelp or Rate my Ratched. I looked over to Cassie. She leapt into action to save me, taking

Nurse Ratched aside for a "chat". She may or may not have used a swear word or two. The head of the CPAP cult backed off. Until she didn't.

All was well and good until Cassie and Dr. Beatles left for the night. Nurse Ratched was wounded from Cassie putting her in her place. She resumed recruiting me for the CPAP cult. In a prior life, she must have been the propaganda official for some totalitarian regime. Or maybe she is the bitter reincarnation of that stupid cat that crashed my bike, which is in the later chapter "Death by Cat". I finally just pretended to read the damn brochure, and that seemed to temporarily satiate her CPAP cult lust. I remember waking up a few times and not only being parched, but my nose was also super dry. There was one of those soft plastic tube thingies pumping oxygen up my nose. I used the call bell to ask for some water and to get rid of the tube. She purposely delayed both bringing me water and helping me get the tube out. I know it was on purpose because I was her only patient. She was literally doing nothing. Ideally, I would have gotten up and grabbed some water myself. But I couldn't raise my arms.

At that time (2009), after a pacemaker install, your arm is put in a tight sling to prevent you raising that arm above chest level. The theory being moving the wrong way could pop your stitches. Or worse, dislodge one of the pacemaker leads, which are anchored in your heart muscles, which are keeping you alive. All this leaves you pretty immobile, so you need a fair bit of help to do even basic things. Things like getting out of bed or getting a tube out of your nose. After maybe my third plea for help (aka her not providing me with proper care), she snarked, "Well maybe if you used a CPAP, you wouldn't have this problem". I was speechless. What was I supposed to do? Order a CPAP on the spot? Does Amazon have a CPAP division with instantaneous delivery? What a nutbar. Morning couldn't come fast enough. I seriously considered reporting Ratched, but I just didn't have the energy. In my subsequent surgeries, they've eliminated the slings, as too many patients ended up with frozen shoulders.

I was released on Friday morning. Cassie came to pick me up and thoughtfully brought a cake for the staff. Except for Nurse Ratched – we should have pied her. With an Ex-Lax pie. We dropped the cake at the nurses' station when a nurse I didn't recognize told me I was a freaking miracle and that I scared the shit out of them. Scared the shit out of them? Pretty sure I had the shit scared out of me, too. Not to flog the proverbial dead horse, but if they had done their jobs and put in the temporary pacemaker, it was likely no shit would have been scared out of anyone. It just seemed like a weird thing to say that bothered me for a long time. As Cassie and I made our way out towards the parking lot, I couldn't believe how weak/trashed/frail/depleted/overwhelmed/emotional/generally dysfunctional I was. Should I really have been released in this condition? Really, should I have been in this condition at all?

LET'S TAKE A SIDE TRIP TO AREA 51

I was simultaneously exhausted and elated just getting to the car. Finally, to be in the sunshine and fresh air for the first time in 10-12 days. Cassie had to run some errands on the way home, so we stopped at the local mall near my place. Trying to take advantage of my newfound freedom, I went into the store with her and quickly realized I needed to be outside again. It was a small store, and it seemed every shopper's goal was to bang into me. I tried walking outside a bit but ran out of gas in about a minute. Thankfully, there was a bench there. In Feb 2018, I asked my current cardiologist, Dr. Pedals (he loves to cycle) if what I experienced that day was normal. He said it wasn't – the large majority of people, even those much older and less healthy than me, come out of surgery relatively functional.

Given Dr. Pedal's revelation, it's time to go full-on cover up/conspiracy theorist on you. We will need all the hospital records to hopefully confirm things, so I don't look like a total nutbar. And I fully accept that many already consider me to be a decorated member of team nutbar. So far, it is mostly circumstantial evidence compiled with the benefit of hindsight. Quick tangent. The word hindsight always makes me laugh because it reminds me of a story by the late observational comedian, David Brenner. At least I hope it is his story. David was on a bus in Philadelphia when a guy in another seat gives him a head nod/glance and says to him "Hey, you done with that?" David didn't know what the guy was talking about, so he followed where the guy's eyes were looking. Brenner realized he was sitting on a newspaper. So he said "Nope, not yet", stood up, turned the page, and sat down again, repeating the act every few minutes until he got off the bus. Hindsight. Get it? I warned you that sometimes I just have to write these things for myself.

Back to the circumstantial evidence that makes me think something was covered up. I know there was a problem in subsequent surgeries that made it really difficult to perform the necessary procedures on me. In surgery one, I 100% went code blue, and they had to abort it. I know I coded because that surgery was performed under a local anesthetic instead of putting me fully to sleep. A week later, they attempted the surgery again. It was almost as bad. When I say bad, I mean stopping in the middle of the second attempt at this procedure and having to videoconference other surgeons around the world during the procedure to figure out workarounds. I was never told exactly what happened until much later and only by happenstance. I had a bunch of repercussions from these procedures that made it necessary to see a vascular surgeon and neurologist. It was via these latter doctors I found out what the problem was.

That's enough Area 51/X-files type thinking for now. We get back to my apartment to find my landlord (who has been fantastic to me in so many ways through a host of medical adventures for which I am eternally grateful) had done some painting, so I couldn't stay at my place until the smell cleared out. A lady from the hood generously offered to let me stay at her place. I thought it would be a nice quiet couple of days. However, it was now Friday evening. What she didn't mention is that she had invited a bunch of friends for Sabbath dinner. She surprised me with a full table of guests, many who visited me the night before the surgery. Thankfully, it was only 10 people or so. But still a crowd to me. Definitely more than I could deal with. They ~~forced me~~ asked me do Kiddush, the ritual blessing of the wine done with Friday night/Sabbath meals. This was the first time the now all too familiar emotional waves hit me. They still hit me to this day (And still in 2022, although to a much lesser degree). I was already drained. Being put on display totally emptied my tank. I suspect this is part of the damage to the vagus nerve, so it now over responds to certain emotional stimuli.

The next day, my host held an open house for people to come visit me. About 100 people came to visit. I was so in shock and depleted that I couldn't extricate myself. I'm sure it looked like I was a willing participant. The reality was I was a total mess. Upon reflection, getting up from the couch and walking up the stairs to hide in my room seems like it should have been a no-brainer. But I just couldn't do it. Cassie and Dr. Beatles came about halfway through and were shocked. Who thinks getting swarmed like this is appropriate for a person just out of surgery? Granted, none of them had a clue what happened to me over the last couple of days. But think about it. If I was still in the hospital, would they have allowed this? Two visitors max normally. At least that's what the signs say.

There was a family who joined the crowd who were in a pretty desperate financial state – I've been there so I get it. I suggested they take some food home. The hostess later shared that she wished I hadn't offered the food. She didn't offer them takeout because she knew something about them that I didn't. It seemed weird to me but hey, everything about these last two weeks was weird. I had bigger fish to fry, even though I am allergic to fish.

THE WISE MEN OF MEDICAL ALERT

A day or two later, I was back at my place, Cassie initiated registering me for a Medical Alert bracelet. Millions of people have them. Let me lay out the collective brainpower for this mission:

Cassie – Multiple bachelor's degrees and ridiculous amounts of professional development,

Me – bachelor's degree, MBA, a few other certifications,

Dr. Beatles – PhD, overall genius.

Overall, a pretty potent group to fill out a simple form on a website. The most challenging part of this exercise should have been choosing the style and colour of the bracelet. At least one would think that. I don't recall what exactly gave us so much grief, but it took us like an hour and a half to get me registered. It was such a comedy of errors that this could have been a Seinfeld episode. Perhaps titled The Medical Alert Nazi – no medical alert bracelets for you!!! Yes, we became temporary members of the Wise Men of Chelm club. Thankfully, we were not afforded permanent member status.

When you get a pacemaker implanted, it needs to be monitored maybe twice a year at the Pacemaker Clinic. Spoiler alert – it's now May 2021. Due to complications, I am at the clinic far too often. However, within a few days of implanting, they want to check you out just to make sure everything works as expected.

What they didn't tell me is I could have done this at the hospital that is significantly closer to where I live. I made the long trek back to the hospital for my appointment, which lasted about seven minutes. I have to admit, how they check it out (formally called interrogating the pacemaker) is pretty Star Treky. Kind of a Bluetooth donut gizmo that is hung over the pacemaker and starts reading the unit. The pacemaker records almost everything, so it shows if you've had fibrillations, if the battery is being drained abnormally and how much juice is left. They can also adjust the pacemaker settings. My pacemaker paces on demand (it reacts to the needs of the body to tell the heart when to beat normally, speed up or slow down). If it doesn't read that it needs to pace, it doesn't and just continues monitoring. As opposed to a pacemaker that is in constant demand at one steady rate. I was being paced at 75%, so my heart's electrical was only telling my heart to beat 25% of the time. As of 2018, I am 100% pacemaker dependent, which means I am being paced 100% of the time as my nerve nodes are completely non-conducting. Or are they? In an October 2020 visit to the pacemaker clinic, something showed up that seemed impossible. Yes, this is a teaser. You'll have to wait for the sequel to find out what happened.

Now that they knew I was safe, Cassie and Dr. Beatles drove back to Montreal to resume their vacation. Even though I had many people to help me out, be it getting lifts, cooking, or just coming for a visit, I felt anxious without my actual family around. I had to go see my family doc Dr. Coif (aka Coiffure) – late 60s and I don't think he's lost a hair in his entire life) to update him and get a replacement cardiologist for Dr. Bland. I've got a great relationship with Coif. Plus, he has an outstanding network of specialists. I'm really fortunate to have him. My friend Hannah Solo (one of the best food smugglers in the galaxy) graciously got me to Dr. Coif's, who quickly got me a much better replacement for Dr. Bland and set me up at the local Pacemaker Clinic.

NOT TO INFLAME THE SITUATION BUT...

I'd had serious body aches, joint-pain, and other physical maladies for years. Nothing that really impaired me, but I knew it was there. Ok, it impaired me. Sometimes I was so sore it was hard getting out of bed. I was probably more acutely aware of this from watching my parents struggling with their various arthritis issues and health issues. Mine? I just racked it up to 30-plus years of hockey, football, rugby and being overweight. I did not know there was a chronic condition called inflammation that was driving all this. Doctors don't tell you something is inflamed unless they are talking about something specific. But body-wide inflammation? Never heard of it until I started Intermittent Fasting in 2018. After rugby games, it was natural to be pretty sore due to all the impact. When I started waking up the day after games and unable to raise my arms because of my shoulders being so sore, I knew it was time to stop and move to mostly non-impact activities. Like beer league hockey. As time passed, it became more apparent that even a full night's sleep wasn't restoring and revitalizing my body. And this was without contact sports. At least three days a week, it was downright painful getting out of bed. Plus, I was generally exhausted. All from what I now know is chronic inflammation. And it was getting worse after my surgery. If it was this bad for me, I can't imagine how painful it has been for my parents. Something pushed me over the inflammation edge. Or had I had it most of my life, getting to the edge gradually?

MY FIRST FULL-ON PUBLIC FLOODING

It's now Wednesday, July 29th, six days after my surgery. Jews have a yearly holiday called Tisha B'Av – the 9th day of the Hebrew month of Av. Like all Jewish days, the day starts at sundown and continues until sundown the next day. The Hebrew calendar runs on a lunar cycle, so its dates aren't anchored to a particular date on the Gregorian calendar. In 2009, Tisha B'Av started at sundown on July 29th. Here, holiday isn't a good descriptor at all. It is a National Day of Mourning so dark that the Rabbis could only describe it by the date, not with a name. Much like 9/11. Many of the great tragedies to befall the Jewish people happened on that date. If it were up to me (and it isn't), I'd remove the date from the calendar, much like many buildings "remove" their 13th floors. During this day, we undertake a 25-hour dry fast, deprive ourselves of routine pleasures, reflect and pray. In fact, Ashkenazi Jews have a 21-day run-up to this day, almost a training camp, where you deny yourself some minor life pleasures to help get you in the mourning/lamenting mindset. Embedded in the 21 days are the (last) nine days, where you don't: eat meat (back in the day it was a celebratory food), dance, listen to live music etc. Growing up, we weren't religious, so I did not know about this day, nor the run-up days existed. As I became more religious, I learned more about the day but as of yet, had never taken part in it. I was still pretty immobile, and I knew I could not make any long treks to synagogue. I also wasn't allowed to do the obligatory fast because I was still pretty fragile. Oh, and I have to eat to take my meds.

My friend Rabbi Restaurant (yes, he is both a Rabbi and a chef) invited me to join him and his father at a small synagogue about 800 metres (about a half mile) from my house. This was usually a six-minute walk for me, but it took 20 plus minutes in my current state. It was also my limit endurance wise. Rabbi Restaurant said would give me a lift home. It was all very surreal to me. I was still in LaLa land to a large degree. Add to that my being totally unfamiliar with the service. Layer on the fact that this was a Sephardic synagogue. Sephardic Jews have different customs than Ashkenazi Jews, so even a regular day service would be different to me. I really had no clue what was going on, except for the reading of the Torah (Bible printed old style on the scrolls). Rabbi Restaurant arranged for me to say the before and after blessing for the first section of the Torah reading, so that I could say an extra blessing of thanks, usually only recited with the Torah reading.

This blessing is said as soon as possible when recovering from an illness or trauma. The idea of the blessing is thanking God for dealing kindly with you, even those that are not really deserving of God's kindness. While I take issue with the part about me not deserving God's kindness, I am all in on the showing gratitude aspect of it. I had never said this prayer before and was having trouble with the Hebrew. Remember, Hebrew had been rudely evicted from my brain from all the concussions, so I was quickly scrambling to learn it phonetically. I knew I was in trouble from the moment I approached the Torah reading area. The emotional flooding started rolling in and I barely made it through the first two blessings. I sputtered and stammered my way through the gratitude blessing and was openly weeping by the time I finished. Those around me, who didn't know me at all, had never seen anyone get so overtly emotional while giving this blessing. It was totally embarrassing. I hated, absolutely hated, being out of control like that. If I thought I had approached my endurance limit walking to the synagogue, I was truly toast now. To this day, these emotional waves come out of nowhere and can hit at anytime. It's a seriously disruptive aspect of one's quality of life. I've even had this happen on job interviews. Needless to say, no one wants a Marketing Director who breaks down when you ask "Tell me something you admire about..." Although now, in 2022, it is far less prevalent. If you want a quality marketing director who might occasionally have a moment, hit me up.

THE RETURN OF DR. PLIÉ

The summer progressed into fall. I tried to go on with my life as best I could, but dammit, it was difficult. I had so many issues affecting me I did not know how to start building myself back up. In fact, I had no clue which issues were actually issues. I was mentally and emotionally paralyzed. The person I really missed the most was my therapist, Dr. Plié, who was off on professional leave. The reality is I didn't know if or when she was coming back. One of the happier days of my life was when Dr. Plié called and said she was coming back to her practice. My response was "Thank God" along with "Do I ever have a story for you!" It took a few weeks to shore up the schedules before we could start working on my triumphant return to, well, ummm, whatever it turned out I was returning to. For a variety of reasons, I wasn't able to deal with the wicked commutes required to getting back to my job as a professor. Add on that my method of teaching was super high energy, which I didn't think I could sustain anymore. Never mind the commute or teaching method. It turns out I was so damaged I've been on permanent disability since my first pacemaker surgery. We focused on getting me functional again. Initially, my thinking was that I'd like to go back to the corporate world. Perhaps as a Director of Marketing. But that's just not going to happen. It would take an extremely benevolent boss to hire me at this point (Dec 2022). What I can handle is hosting The

Dead Man Walking Podcast or the odd speaking engagement. So if you are some corporate entity looking to bring in a kick-ass speaker or to sponsor some great content, hit me up. You'll get a big bang for your buck.

Dr. Plié and I started working together again in Jan 2010. Something we worked a lot on was improving my non-verbal skills so I could better understand social cues and situations. Because of all my trauma, I had regressed in some areas I had previously made progress in, so that needed addressing. Of course, we also needed to address the myriad of PTSD/Post-concussion afflictions that were now layered on top of my previous challenges. There is no established treatment plan for this, as each person's afflictions are different. A challenging situation for both of us. In March 2018, I asked Dr. Plié what she recalled from those early sessions and her reaction to my story. The Doc just shared with me that when we resumed our sessions, she took a while to get back in the groove, so she'd need to check her notes. I feel truly awful. I wasn't more aware and sensitive to her situation. Her situation being that when you take a long work sabbatical, it isn't easy for many to reacclimate to the job. Especially one as intense as psychiatry. I hold her in such high esteem that I never considered her not hitting the ground running. I missed big on that one. Improving my situational awareness is just something I have to continue working on, I guess. She always took copious amounts of notes, which is great because referring to them could help easily overcome the gaps, both mine and hers. Mostly she remembers being shocked. Utterly shocked. I was shell-shocked. I guess, to a degree, I still am. Which Dr. Plié says is part of the reason the emotional waves keep rolling in. Despite all the work we've done and the fact all my standard health markers (blood work, blood pressure) are good, this evil still lives inside me. And it was just bidding its time, plotting its next emergence.

There is also general anxiety constantly running in the background. Often, it doesn't even try to hide. It's just there. Even now, as I write this in August 2020, every time something seems off health or emotionally, my first thought is something is going wrong with the pacemaker again (and it often is). In fact, my cardiologist, Dr. Pedals eventually told me that if I feel off beyond something obvious like a cold, just go to emergency. Much like seeing a duck floating in a pond. It looks so peaceful and effortless, but underneath the water, those little duck legs (or my brain) are churning furiously. It's really hard for me to identify when I am just having a normal human hiccup or if something is actually happening to me physically. Every time I have, say, a bit of dizziness or lose my balance or my vision gets blurry for whatever reason, the anxiety comes forward and mocks me with "Ha-ha, your heart is stopping again!" I can't tell you how much energy this drains from a person. Some events are worse than others. For example, on June 23/2010, I thought I was having a brainquake again. I was vibrating. It looked to me like the walls were waving (It turns out they were). It was so unnerving that I called 911 but couldn't get through, which significantly increased my level of being unnerved.

My symptoms abated. I calmed down. One of my safety clues is that I wasn't pouring sweat like other times. Soon after, I went online to learn that Toronto had experienced a mild earthquake, which was why the 911 system was swamped. For once, my symptoms were totally external and had nothing to do with my heart. This is pure speculation on my part, but I'd like to think if I wasn't in this constant state of anxiety, I would have realized it was a minor earthquake in the moment. That I wasn't having a brainquake and the walls really were moving. So be forewarned earthquakes, I am on to you. You bastards won't fool me a second time.

MY SUN-BLEACHED BONES

We're going to take a jump forward in the time machine to August 2010. We finally get to move forward to something positive and happy. It was time for my nephew's Bar Mitzvah in beautiful Nova Scotia. A lot of my family was going to attend, several whom we hadn't seen since we were teens. An added plus was the parents being up to travel health-wise. It was off to Halifax we went for a much-needed five-day vacation. Although I love family time, it can also be a stressful time because of family dynamics. Dr. Plié and I always try to strategize some coping techniques to help me survive these adventures. All went well for the most part. There were no obvious conflicts or blow-ups. We even got to spend some time at Peggy's Cove. It is one of Nova Scotia's treasures, a small fishing village with an awesome lighthouse. Very touristy. Search Engine it. Or better yet, go visit. Tell them I sent you.

To me, the best part of Peggy's Cove is not wandering from shop-to-shop looking at all the art or locally produced trinkets. Warning - bring deep pockets. Or at least a credit card with a good limit on it. This stuff ain't cheap. It is a tourist trap, after all. The little ice cream shop, however, is totally worth the extra. Or even the Lighthouse. In my view, the unquestioned best thing about Peggy's Cove is being able to walk out onto the huge outcropping of rock that is exposed to the pounding Atlantic Ocean. Search pictures of that too. Or watch a video. It's amazing. I find the power of the waves crashing fascinating. It is Mother Nature at her best. It's not a straight walk from the parking lot to wherever on the rock you decide to venture to. The distance is probably 300-500 metres as the crow flies but about twice that when you navigate all the fissures and climbing. I had started out with my brother's family then went off on my own. After some time, I decided to head back to the lighthouse. I'm not sure what happened but some aspect of PTSD/Post-concussion kicked in and my brain suddenly withheld all my balance and depth perception capabilities.

I was frozen. I couldn't tell if something was a little crack I could step over or jump across or whether it was 4-5 feet across. I also couldn't tell if it was a two-foot drop or 20 feet. I was on the verge of panicking. Then I had a moment of clarity. Just sit down – nothing could happen to me if I just sat down, right? Besides, there were people around and someone would notice me. Or they would eventually find my sun-bleached bones. One or the other. After some time, I tried playing a game of chess with the rocks and crevices, making moves and counter moves to inch my way back. This strategy allowed me to minimize falling, but was taking an awfully long time. I don't know exactly how long it took me to slither back, but I am guessing at least an hour. Two slithers forward, three slithers back and/or to the side. I was exhausted by the time I got to relatively solid ground. PTSD/Post-concussion makes a horrible companion, and an even worse travelling companion. That being said, I am looking forward to my next visit to Peggy's Cove. It's that good.

When I got back to Toronto, Dr. Coif and I decided getting into the Cardiac Rehab program would be really beneficial for me. It's a structured fitness and education program for, you guessed it, people with cardiac issues. Even if it was a ridiculous effort to get there and back – about 1.5 hours each way. No one told me I was eligible to take the Wheel Trans system. Wheel Trans is basically a subsidized cab that takes passengers door-to-door for the price of a bus ticket. Although I don't think they use tickets or tokens anymore. The Rehab program didn't start up again until October, so my only real rehab was walking and any learning I did on my own. The program's intake appointment finally arrives, and we have to do two 3-hour intake sessions on diet and exercise that pretty much bored every person there to tears. I was far and away the youngest participant. I suspect a few were easily 40 years older than me. Not exactly a high energy event. What I also quickly learned in the orientations is that every expert in there had a divergent view of what constituted good health and proper rehab. One told me to lift weights. The next said no weights, just use resistance bands. No, not resistance bands – do yoga. No, you can't do yoga. If you invert yourself, it will mess up your pacemaker. I called Dr. Pedals, who nearly dropped the phone laughing about the yoga prophecy. He said, "the reason you have the pacemaker is so you CAN do things like yoga and be alive. Roller coasters and things like that may cause massive sudden shifts in blood pressure, so stay away from those. But yoga? Enjoy". I was hoping they would just let me go into the Rehab gym and do my thing on my own. But no such luck. I tried the home exercise program, but to be honest, it was really uninspiring working out alone. It reminded me too much of the old calisthenics programs Mom and the ladies used to watch on TV, like Jack LaLanne. I think there were a number of exercise peeps on TV in the mid 60's, but his is the only name I recall. Coincidentally, I had my weekly scheduled video call with my mother today (July 2020). She's in a nursing home and needs an attendant with her to operate the phone, so thus, the scheduling.

I asked if she remembered doing these exercise classes and she replied smilingly, "Yep, once a week. We rotated houses – exercised and then we ate". For exercise, I went back to the old standby – my mountain bike. And quickly recognized how out of shape I had become. And more importantly, how hilly Toronto is compared to Winnipeg. Thank God for gears. Even with gears, cycling was still quite the challenge.

SOME JEWISH PERSPECTIVE ON DEATH

Much of mainstream society has this idyllic vision of heaven. I don't know where the idea of floating around on clouds dressed in white, with all of us having wings, came from. I know the Cherubs on the original Ark of the Covenant had wings, but they weren't angels. Jewish liturgy doesn't seem to have a lot of commentaries regarding what your soul does once it gets cleared into the world to come. Although some stories talk about those who are "worthy" getting to attend the heavenly equivalents of Masterclasses, which are all the rage right now. Except these are the ultimate Masterclasses – taught by God, Moses, Aaron etc. What the commentaries do talk about is the entrance requirements. Which are quite different than St. Peter meeting you at a gate. Although I do like many of the jokes that have come from St. Peter manning the gate. What's my favourite one? Glad you asked. It helps to be a hockey fan for this one. Gentleman gets admitted to heaven and St. Peter is giving him the grand tour of pretty much anything one could desire. As they proceed, the guy hears the familiar sound of skate blades cutting the ice along with slap shots and pucks hitting goalposts. Obviously, this guy is Canadian. They wander towards a skating rink and see someone gliding around effortlessly. The gentleman says to St. Peter "Impressive, who is he?" St. Peter responds "Him, oh. That's just

God. He likes to think he's Wayne Gretzky". But alas, once again I have taken you to TangentVille.

Warning - Please consult with your local Orthodox Rabbi (LOR) before taking what I have been taught/researched/understand as the singular way to interpret our learnings. There is no singular way. As they say, put four rabbis in a room, you get significantly more than four opinions. Traditional Judaism believes that while you are alive, your soul is bound to your physical body. When one dies, the glue holding the soul to the body dissipates. The soul loses its anchor, but still tries to stay with the body. It is lost, or maybe more accurately, rudderless and in an agitated state, until the burial. There are a few rituals we do to help the soul lessen its agitation. Or at least we hope these rituals work. There is no way to really know. First, we never leave the deceased alone. Second, we have people saying psalms (prayers) in their vicinity 24/7. And third, we bury them asap to allow that last earthly bond to be broken and send the soul to the world to come. Or to however you define heaven or the heavenly court.

Now here is where I think it gets interesting. The Jewish tradition is that upon arrival, God meets us and asks between three-to-six questions, depending on your situation:

Were your business dealings be'Emunah (honest)?

Did you fix Itim (times) for Torah (Old Testament) learning?

Did you engage in Peru u'Rvu (Chosen)? For males only. The commandment is for men to procreate, not women. Yeah, kinda difficult to figure out, but it's there in the Bible.

Did you anticipate Yeshu'ah (salvation) aka repent?

Did you delve deeply into Chachmah (the wisdom of the sages)?

Did you understand one matter through another to attain greater Da'as/General Wisdom]?

How you answer these questions plays a big part in what happens next at your "trial". The angels split up into teams, shirts and skins. Ooops. I meant prosecutors and defence. Then they go to battle to help decide if your good deeds outweigh your bad and by how much. This is all to decide how much time you spend in (hard G) Gehenim. Not that it's a big deal, but people are always arguing how to pronounce Gif – is it a hard G or is it a "J" sound like Jif? Ah, first world problems. A good way to describe Gehenim is it is a combination of spiritual soul washing/scrubbing and refurbishing centre. Again, repurposing is good for the environment. The truly righteous skip this step, so the better you are, the fewer months you spend there. It's believed the maximum time you can spend here is 12 months. That's if you are evil personified. The large majority of people do less than 12 months. During the traditional mourning periods, children mourn and say prayers for their parents for 11 months. No one mourns and prays for the full 12 months. I did it for my father in 2015-16 and I am doing it for my mother, who passed in June 2022. I also have done this for friends and relatives who don't have family to take on this spiritual obligation. Rumour is that getting scrubbed is not a pleasant experience. Although we can't really confirm this, can we?

CLEOPATRA ON RESURRECTION

Probably like you, I have so many questions about this. Once you are scrubbed, are you deemed one of the truly righteous? If not, what happens to you? I know we believe in resurrection. At Mt. Sinai, God gave the Jews the Ten Commandments a few times. The first two times were orally. The voice of God was so powerful that it scared the souls out of everyone there. Moses had to ask God to resurrect them. Not just once, but twice! We also believe when the Messiah comes, the righteous will be resurrected. Which leads to question one: What gets you into the righteous club to qualify for resurrection? Which brings me to question two, asked by one of our significant sources of Jewish thought (insert sarcasm here). Queen Cleopatra. Yep. That Cleopatra, Queen of the Nile, who some say invented lipstick. The original influencer. The Kim Kardashian of her time. She asked one of the great sages of the times, Rabbi Meir (pronounced May-er) if when the righteous are resurrected, will they be wearing their clothes? Given her interest in makeup and fashion, I can see why she would be so concerned about clothing. And it hints at her desire to become one of the righteous. But let's face it – she had a long road to travel. Afterall, she arranged the deaths of both her brother and sister. And allegedly was having an affair with said brother. Let's put that aside and get back to why Cleopatra was interested in the Jewish learnings at all. The Egyptians have their own really strong death and after death culture. Let's ignore the fact that Jews are generally not buried in their clothes but in a simple shroud. I also don't know how Cleopatra and Rabbi Meir knew each other or how they were communicating. To preserve the story, I'm going to totally ignore the fact that Queen Cleo died roughly 300 years before Meir was born. Meir was sort of the John Lennon or Albert Einstein of the great rabbis of the time. Few could keep up with his thought processes. Maybe they met on a WhatsApp time-traveling Hieroglyphic thread, became friendly through that, and messaged regularly? Or via some sort of pyramid scheme? Sorry, that joke was just so obvious.

Some extra background on Jewish traditions and learning is required here. In addition to the Ten Commandments/Bible that God gave Moses at Mt. Sinai, Jews believe that God also gave Moses the Mishna, also known as the Oral Tradition. That is, a secondary set of laws to explain the commandments more deeply (For those of you keeping score, there are 613 of them embedded within the original ten commandments). Examples that may be familiar to you are "Keeping the Sabbath" or the dietary laws of "Keeping Kosher". Factoid: The actual commandments are to guard and to remember the Sabbath. Regardless, the Bible never explains what keeping, guarding, or remembering the Sabbath entails, but we know what it entails since Jews have been "Keeping the Sabbath" since, well, since there have been Jews. The same is with keeping Kosher. Both these seemingly simple concepts are actually quite complex to execute. Jews learn how to keep these laws through the Oral Tradition.

The second component of this aspect of learning is called The Gemara (again, hard G). It means "to study". The Gemara takes the Oral Tradition laws (the Mishna) and breaks them down into dozens of categories, which the ancient Rabbis discuss, debate, analyzed and explain. When I started learning Gemara, I was quite stunned how smart and how much wisdom existed thousands of years ago. Six years later, I am still awed by the depths of their understanding. The combination of the Mishna and Gemara is called The Talmud, but colloquially, we now use Gemara and Talmud interchangeably.

Back to Cleo and Rabbi Meir. The Gemara, in the book titled Sanhedrin (page 90b) discusses this exchange of ideas. Queen Cleopatra asked Rabbi Meir "I know that the dead will revive, for it is written "And they [sc.the righteous] shall [in the distant future] blossom forth out of the city [Jerusalem] like the grass of the earth. But when they arise, shall they arise nude or in their garments?"" Rabbi Meir replied "Thou mayest deduce by an a fortiori argument [the answer] from a wheat grain: if a grain of wheat, which is buried naked, sprouteth forth in many robes, how much more so the righteous, who are buried in their raiment!" So, there you have it. I do not know why R. Meir apparently spoke in some variant of Shakespearean English. The actual point is that you shy, righteous people don't have to worry about modesty when you are resurrected. You will be fully clothed. We can only guess as to whether you are assigned a personal stylist and get to choose your clothes. Oh, and I still do not know what happens next.

You can contrast this with one of the mainstream concepts of what happens when you die, which is the premise of many near death experience stories. And I am not dismissing anyone else's experience. Because I've also had out-of-body type experiences where I've been looking at myself and at others through a detached third-party perspective. I suspect I was clinically dead during those out-of-body episodes. Or perhaps I might have been dreaming or maybe in a fever state. Or maybe it was something else entirely. It is too hard to say. However, what can't be disputed is that I've experienced these things in the past. It would be disingenuous of me to dismiss others' claims about their experiences. Such as those who report seeing lights, people calling to them, or a sense of calmness.

Although it might make a better story, I can't make stuff up. There was no out-of-body, come to the light events for me - no bright lights, no warm glow, no one calling me to come to the other side. Just dead. Twenty times and not once did I get anything resembling being called to the other side or the light. I feel kind of ripped off. But I had a Fred kind of death, so why would I expect anything normal?

THE NOT SO SCIENTIFIC/PERSONAL PERSPECTIVE

There is no definitive way to explain my not experiencing any come to the light episodes or experiences in the same vein that others have reported. Not everyone has them. I am going to propose that all my brain trauma, past and present, broke my spiritual radar. I know everyone is different. Even though I go to daily prayers as often as possible, do my bible study dutifully and observe (to the level I am able) the Jewish customs and traditions, I don't seem to get that spiritual pump/connection/passion/feelings that others seem to get. Maybe I'm just trying or hoping to jam my spiritual square peg into the proverbial (see what I did there?) holy round hole. Maybe it will change in the future. Your guess is as good as mine.

BABY YOU CAN DRIVE MY CAR

Speaking of guesses, people have asked me what has kept me going. How am I so resilient? What drives me? I think all are good questions. Not questions I know how to answer easily. I think we all have some level of resiliency gene built in that has allowed humanity and the world at large to evolve and adapt for millions of years. It sort of runs in the background, runs on its own and we don't realize we have this capability. Even under stress or duress, when we are being resilient, we don't have thoughts that pat ourselves on the back for being resilient any more than we have a conscious thought we need to keep breathing. And yes, I know you are all going to be conscious of your need to breathe now. Sorry. I won't mention being aware of your tongue, either. During the horrors of the world wars, post 9/11, during the Covid pandemic, I've heard no one saying or quoted that they are being resilient. It's just a state of being.

Resiliency, drive, never quit, overcoming adversity. However you name it, it likely has roots in the nature versus nurture conversation. Both play a factor. I believe a lot of my resilience came from watching my parents have all their issues. Despite that, they just kept chugging along. I wasn't actively thinking, "Oh, so Mom and Dad are outstanding models of resiliency. I need to learn and apply this". Nor did they ever say to me you need to do A, B, and C to be resilient or to overcome adversity. It was just being uploaded into my damaged brain, to be used whenever my brain started healing and processing properly. Speaking of my damaged brain, I believe trauma and injury just activates our body to seek out solutions to get back to a healthy state. From the days of my original brain trauma, I was put into some kind of seek, research, repair, upgrade, repeat mode. Was it always moving in a linear fashion? Nope. It moved at the pace it was capable of. For me, that seems to upcycle in my 30s.

That being said, there seem to be multiple spectrums of resilience. Some are more resilient for some things, some less. Some have really limited areas of resilience. And we have different levels of resilience at different points in our lives. Some can only be resilient if they have a goal. Say, playing in the NFL. They will do anything and commit every resource possible to achieving that goal. And if they don't make it, they often flounder. Maybe they just burned out their resiliency gene or superpower. I don't know. We see this in the corporate world, in relationships, all around us. You could be looking at someone being resilient beyond their wildest dreams right now and have no clue. Nor do they. I have a couple of MBA buddies who have done very well in the corporate world. If you ask them for any secrets of their success, what drives them, how they overcome adversity, it is like watching athletes being interviewed. Very cliched. "Gotta take it one play at a time, take advantage of the opportunities, give 110%, work smarter, not harder, sacrifice for the team". They cannot articulate what gives them that unique drive to succeed, to be better, to overachieve. Much like seeing someone whom you think has a perfect life, but little do you know. They are fighting tremendous battles on many fronts, most of which we cannot even comprehend.

Another thing I noticed about these questions. What exactly do they think I am being resilient or having this amazing drive for? I never thought to ask for a clarification. Not dying? I think we all have that superpower. Was I not supposed to call the ambulances or have surgeries? Having a life? Aren't we here to have lives, relationships, purpose, serve God (for those of you into that sort of mindset?) I don't know how to give up on that. Maybe they mean writing this book? This one I can answer. It started as a small exercise, then as I went along, it became more important. I saw the self-publishing world evolve and a good number of people being successful. Plenty were failing, just like traditional publishing. And I met a few people who had become very successful self-publishing. Combined with my obvious gifts, story telling and writing, I said "Why not me? I have a great story that needs to be told". Layering on that, it became apparent that because of my health issues, I could never hold a traditional job again. I needed an income. Somehow, I was going to turn this small project into my livelihood. And reclaim the years that had been stolen from me. And I can't forget, Mr. Calcutta (you'll meet him later), said I have an angel watching over me. To which Mrs. Calcutta chimed in, "An Angel? He must have an entire team!" I can't argue with that.

SOME OF THE MORE OBVIOUS
ONGOING ISSUES

It's probably not so abnormal to not be able to pinpoint all the ongoing issues when one has been through all the trauma I just went through. Aided by the lenses I can look through as time has passed, here are just a few of things that went additionally wonky on me because of the Traumatic Brain Injuries (TBIs) added on to my previous Acquired Brain Injuries (ABIs).

While I've been essentially legally blind in my left eye since birth, I had a certain level of peripheral/blurred vision I could count on to give me a minimal degree of sight and spatial awareness. But mostly only if I close my right eye as my brain can't process the visual input from both eyes at the same time. You know when you go for an eye test, and they put that paddle thing in front of your eye to block what it sees? When they do that for me, my right eye is so dominant that if I don't close my right eye, I mostly see the paddle even though it is my left eye looking at the screen. I've never been given a satisfactory answer what causes this. Nonetheless, it seems to have gone to a lower level of blind since all this head trauma. Whatever activity I engage in, be it driving, walking, riding a bike, etc., I can't trust a single shoulder check to make sure it is safe to proceed. It often takes two, three, or four checks (especially at night), to make sure I am safe to proceed. Sometimes, depending on a variety of factors, I may need to pull over so I can do a full head turn to make sure I can safely proceed.

To the best of my recollection, I've never been afraid of heights or ledges or falling. Now, I am. Even with all my collapses, I've mostly fallen from 4 to 5 feet at the most. Certainly not from any great heights or edges of buildings. The PTSD/Concussion Gremlins have now deemed that this shall now be an ongoing issue for me. Even watching TV or a movie, if a character is in a precarious position (say, a ledge of a building), it makes me physically uncomfortable. I would say it's like a flooding event with some terror added. In everyday life, it makes things like subway stations some of my least favourite destinations. Some have entry stairs of three or four floors, so looking down to the bottom doesn't elicit feelings of joy in me. Nor do the platforms, which are slightly slanted towards the tracks for drainage. There are days I get sensory overload and it feels more like the slant of a playground slide. It feels like I am going to lose my footing and slide into the abyss. Despite seeing 100s of people around me who this wasn't happening to.

The TBIs also negatively influenced my depth perception and balance. Particularly going down sets of stairs. This just reminded me I used to have a babysitter named Mrs. Stairs – It was an up and down relationship. Oddly, she had a sister-in-law named Mrs. Stares. I don't think I saw eye-to-eye with her. Ok, back to my balance issues – stumbling going down sets of stairs. I find it interesting that I have no issues going up stairs, but down the stairs – Yeesh! There have been several times where complete strangers at the subway stations have grabbed me, saving me from a tumble down the stairs. Of course, they often ask "Are you drunk?" or "What are you on, buddy?". I don't blame them. Embarrassingly, I try to explain I have a brain injury that gives me problems and thank them for helping me out. I'd guess it is 50/50 as to who believes me versus who thinks I am some sort of substance abuser.

Soon after I realized Hebrew had been evicted from my brain, I also realized that both my general reading comprehension and reading speed were way down. I've confirmed this with periodic testing. I don't know how I knew this, but it seemed to me that getting these benchmarks normal again would be a major component of my recovery. Forcing myself to read content that normally wasn't in my wheelhouse was the key. I tried reading all sorts of stuff that I normally would not read. I have since learned this activates neuroplasticity, a fancy word for resetting one's neural/brain functions. Additionally, I was taught another Jewish concept: God gives us the cures before he gives us the disease. That is likely how I knew to read outside what I normally read. And if describing God with the pronoun "he" triggers you, feel free to use whatever pronoun de-triggers you. I'm just here to tell a story.

Just communicating became a challenge. Although, upon reflection, I think I was more aware of this than those I was speaking with. I often couldn't come up with the words I wanted to say. The pauses seemed like five, ten seconds or more, but probably were no where near that. The same with slurring my words, especially when I finally found the words and tried to insert them into my sentences. It seemed terribly obvious to me, but mostly not to others. Unless they were just being super polite and not mentioning it. Although there were sometimes that even with my lower skill level of reading non-verbal cues, I could see people's reactions. I know I was slurring big time and had to repeat/clarify what I was trying to say.

One of the strangest after effects of all this was the apparent near total reversal of my circadian rhythms or circadian clock. This is our internal process that basically regulates our sleep/wake cycles and is based on a 24-hour schedule. For most of my life, I was a reasonably early riser and could go to sleep at 11 PM, give or take. Like most people, I could get up an extra hour early if I wanted to get to the gym or work or airport if need be. As well, I could stay up later if called for. However, this head trauma totally messed up my clock. Without a sleep aid, I rarely fell asleep before 2-3 AM. And even if I did, I was wide awake after two hours of sleep. Which meant I was not waking until 10-11 AM. It really makes it hard to get anything done when you are not on the same schedule as most of your community. Thankfully (as of 2021), Intermittent Fasting, which you will learn about later in the book, plus neuroplasticity, has gotten my circadian clock almost back to normal.

If you end up in a situation like me, first, I wish the best for you. It seems the biggest take away for me is how our views of what science and medicine can do for us have been totally distorted. We have grossly unrealistic expectations. From Star Trek to all the modern medical shows, there are unrealistic ideals of how hospital and medical teams work. Rarely are there wait times, and if there are, someone just calls someone else and magically, everyone waiting gets transported to another area of the hospital for immediate care. In those shows, almost everyone gets fixed, no scars, no side or residual effects. The idea that every doctor and nurse is almost singularly working on you, or your case/issue, is just not real. That every resource needed is available just isn't a reality. That just because you ask for something doesn't mean anyone will hear you or that you will get it. If you have any type of faith, it will be tested.

WELCOME TO 2013
THE FALL I DIED 20 TIMES
(AKA 20 MORE SHADES OF COGNITIVE BIAS)

I guess this is kind of what it is like to be one of those TV shows either critics like and the viewers don't support, or the viewers love the show, and the critics hate it. The show has the season one finale but no one on the show knows what the future holds. Maybe this was not just the season finale but also the series finale? Do we get another shot, and if we do, will there be cast changes, storylines altered, location changes along with so many other factors? Or will it be relatively smooth sailing? Well, from the cardiologists' perspectives, I had a functioning pacemaker. I was definitely renewed for the next season and beyond with no constraints. I subsequently learned there are a few constraints – no riding on roller coasters and Canadian Blood Services no longer allows me to donate blood (In December 2021, I convinced them it was safe for me to donate again. Victory!!! Please donate and help save a life.) Alas, there were factors beyond the life saving miracle of the pacemaker at play. And then the miracle turned on me. This might sound familiar - my name is Fred Rutman. And do I have another story for you.

Upon reflection, I now realize that Season 2 of *The Summer I Died Twenty Times* started in mid-August 2013 and not in October, as we initially thought. The doctors and I simply misdiagnosed the symptoms I experienced as over exertion while I was cycling. I know, right? Shocker. I was on the long road back from the Summer of Death 2009 tour recovering from all the Post-concussion syndromes and just being really beat up. Yep, four years later and was just back to maybe 80% of what I was. I was working hard on my fitness, primarily by cycling. I noticed when I stopped after a bit of a longer ride (well, longer for me), I was either dizzy and/or a bit wobbly. I needed to get off the bike and sit in the shade, totally depleted. I mean your phone battery reading 1% levels of depleted. The doctors thought it was from exertion. To quote 45, yep, we were bigly wrong.

THE 2013 TOUR DE SPLAT

That old saying that things are right in front of you, yet you still can't see the forest through the trees is pretty spot on. I was on a particularly (again, for me) long bike ride and I was feeling pretty pleased with myself. It was a warm day. I had done a couple of hills I wasn't able to conquer previously and rode to a new neighbourhood. I was starting home and took a shortcut through a funky little park. I was following the path and saw something ahead. I don't have the greatest vision and couldn't tell what it was. Perhaps an injured animal, a jacket, a bag of garbage? As I got closer, I could see that someone dumped a pile of sand on the pavement. "Who does that?" I thought, quickly followed by, "Big deal. Easy peasy. I'm on a mountain bike. I can plow through that".

The next thing I know, I hit the pile of sand and suddenly had no power. I stopped dead (no pun intended) in my tracks and toppled over. I tumbled so quickly that I had no chance of getting my hands off the handlebars or my feet out of the pedal traps. When I came to, I was sore but not really damaged. I suspect I was out for a while and figured I must have hit my head. There was no reason to think otherwise. Then I began to recognize what had happened. Another subtle brainquake and fireworks display. Unlike all the other times, at least I was wearing a helmet this time.

But I should have paid attention to my Spidey Sense. Something was up.

But what that was, I didn't know. I sat in the shade for half an hour or so until I felt steady again. My breathing slowed, and I stopped sweating, both of which I attributed to having been exercising hard on a fairly warm day. I made it home without further incident, feeling pretty pleased overall with my effort and having stretched myself. I was making progress. Being a typical guy, I almost immediately forgot about the episode and what happened to me.

Things seemed to progress normally through September, except for the recurring dizzy/wobbly symptoms that the medical team just attributed to exercising hard/blood sugar issues through the warm weather. After all, I was also diabetic, so wonky blood sugar levels are to be expected. The pacemaker checkups showed nothing, except that my heart was becoming more dependent on the pacemaker. I was now using the pacemaker 90% of the time. I was feeling good, my Post-concussion symptoms were much improved, and I enrolled in an Advanced Digital Marketing course to further gauge my readiness to re-enter the world of the working. It was at this point I became a full participant in Fred's Season 2 of *The Summer I Died Twenty Times*. AKA the 2013 Autumn of Death tour. If you thought Fred's 2009 Summer of Death Tour was ridiculous, you ain't seen nothing yet.

I know I was making progress with trying to improve my learning, diet, and exercising. As part of the Cardiac Rehab program, you can get an annual stress test. That should be an excellent benchmark. At this point (November 2020), I am currently overdue for one, so maybe after all this Covid stuff passes, I can get one. I suspect there will be a long waiting list. Back to 2013. You aren't supposed to exercise before the test, so I threw my bike on the convenient bike racks on the bus, then made my way to the Rehab Centre. Those bike racks on the bus are a great tool. If only someone could figure out how to add these to the subway cars as well. It takes 90 minutes to Rehab by bus, 40 minutes by bike. October 7, I sign all the stress test paperwork and waivers and go for it. I was pleased with my results - I came out upper average in fitness for my age group. I think my age category is listed as "alta kaker", a Yiddish term for old fart. Upon reflection, it was not a good idea to ride the bike home from the stress test. Of course, it was uphill and against a 65 kph/35 mph wind all the way. Then again, it seems almost every time I ride, it is uphill and against the wind. Even when I am going downhill. One time it was so windy I joked to a buddy I was surprised the wind didn't push the light back into my bike lights.

THE START OF THE 2013 FALL DEATH TOUR

It was around 7 a.m. Saturday morning, October 19, 2013. I had an unusually fitful sleep with weird dreams. I got out of bed. Normally, if you only get a few hours of sleep, you expect to be somewhat tired. This wasn't a normal tired. I drove right past overly tired and straight to exhausted. I thought I would try reading on the couch; hopefully, I'd fall asleep for an hour or so, feel better, then go to synagogue for services. I started reading and then just like Fred's 2009 Summer of Death Tour, the extra strength brainquake hit, followed by the brilliant fireworks display and everything that went along with it was pounding at me. I was so confused. I wasn't exactly sure what was going on because my heart couldn't be stopping – I had a fully functioning pacemaker. And pacemakers don't fail. Right?

I got up and tried to make it to, well, I wasn't exactly sure where I'd make it to. There wasn't really a plan. I remember the brainquake hit again, followed by me collapsing, and slamming my head into the flat screen TV (may it rest in pieces). More fireworks, more brainquakes, then a moment of clarity. I need to get to the hospital, I thought. Good thing I can just hop the bus to the Subway, which goes almost door-to-door to the hospital. Then I started looking for my subway tokens. Ok, so obviously, the moment of clarity wasn't so clear. Another brainquake or two followed by the fireworks.

I finally got it together to a degree, managing to call 911 (at least I was together enough to remember the number). I recall more than a few TV shows where characters comically couldn't grasp how 911 works. In an episode of Home Improvement, Tim Allen's Tim Taylor character calls the operator and says "Operator - what's the number for 911?" followed by "Geez, operator. Can you slow it down? I'm trying to take notes here". At least I was outperforming Tim. I finally got to talk to someone in the ambulance department. I tried explaining what was happening to me but really couldn't articulate it, which frustrated the 911 operator. Further, the brainquakes and fireworks hit again mid-conversation. I could finally bluster that I was experiencing the same symptoms that lead me to need the original pacemaker. The operator said it was impossible, pacemakers don't fail. I know, right? But yet, here I am. Then the brainquakes and fireworks happened again. I am not sure how long I was gone, but the first thing I heard was the 911 operator screaming frantically, telling me the EMTs were on the way.

Thinking this was going to be another long-term adventure, I managed to pack a travel bag and my electronics (gotta stay connected after all), then made my way out to the front porch. As the EMTs approached, they went from walking to a full-on sprint. I guess I wasn't looking so good. No messing around. Strapped me on the stretcher and got me loaded up. I mentioned I was also feeling nauseous, which was a new symptom. They gave me the BCU – Barf Containment Unit. Then, with no warning, I projectile vomited. The BCU didn't stand a chance. There was vomit everywhere, especially on me. We tried to clean me up the best we could, which required removing my monitor leads and the blood pressure cuff. You know what that means. More brainquakes and fireworks. Getting toward the hospital, one of the EMTs said she remembered me from my previous death tour. I filled her in somewhat on what eventually happened with me. "That's the most insane story I've ever heard. Don't worry. We'll take good care of you". she commented, adding it was her first day back after maternity leave. I joked she wasn't pinning that on me. They got me in to the hospital and parked me in the hallway. I seemed stable, so they went to update the triage nurse. Which turned out to have been a less than great idea.

WELCOME TO THE HOTEL RESUSCITATION (INSERT GUITAR SOLO HERE)

My apologies to any band who may or may not have a similar song title or lyrics. Another brainquake and the resultant fireworks. When I opened my eyes, there was a group of non-hospital people just staring at me like they had seen an alien emerge from inside me. "What the fuck just happened to you?" one blurted out. I guess I had some seizure-like body movements during these episodes, and it looked pretty freaky. It's understandable they were freaked out, but geez, maybe let someone know this is going on? I'm not on a gurney in ER for no reason. I probably should have asked the EMTs what happens when the brainquakes and fireworks hit, as they were the only others to witness this, but I was in no condition to make a to-do list. Suddenly, a group of nurses swooped in and rushed me into the Resus (Resuscitation) Room. It's not a room you want frequent flier points for. They cut my puke-soaked shirt off me. An internist came in and asked me a million questions and had no clue. They were doing the usual ECGs, blood work etc. I am quite sure I had a couple more episodes (Are we up to 20 yet? Must be pretty close).

Finally (and by finally, I mean like 4 or 5 hours later), an actual cardiologist wanders in. I think it was Dr. Angio, who oversaw my angiogram in 2009. He instructs whomever to get the magnet and hold it over my pacemaker to reset it. It was not your standard fridge magnet, probably 4 pounds. After holding this bolder on me for maybe half an hour, the nurses decided holding the magnet on me wasn't the best use of their time. They wrapped me in some hospital version of duct tape or something like it to keep the magnet in place so they wouldn't have to hold it. The cardiologist returns and asks if anyone called the technician from the pacemaker company.

You could have heard a pin drop, with everyone looking completely stunned. "Come on. No one thought to call the tech?" Finally, the cardiologist makes the call himself and we find the technician is on a case about seven hours out of town, so he will get here as soon as he can. Later, the internist comes to me with a big grin on his face and says, "I've been doing this for 20 years and had never seen a suspected pacemaker fail. And I for sure had no clue there was a pacemaker technician to call. You learn something new every day!" He seemed quite pleased with himself. Like this was a good thing, that neither he (nor the rest of the emergency staff) knew about these potential life-saving tools. I encountered this guy again at the end of 2018. An odd duck, to say the least.

Finally, the pacemaker technician arrived. He looks as fried as I imagined my pacemaker is. Easily on hour 16 of his day, tons of highway driving through crappy weather and probably not functioning at his peak. After a few minutes, the cardiologist comes in and asks him to interrogate (retrieve and analyze the data from) the pacemaker. Techie tells the doc that using the magnet probably wiped the data (not true, I later find out). Also, he has to remove the magnet and the 40 feet of tape they used to keep the magnet on my beastly hairy body. Ex-freaking-scruciating!!! Probably not as awful as the chest waxing scenes in the movie 40-Year-Old Virgin, but I was already so beat up. The interrogation was, of course, totally inconclusive. And I finally recognized that

I should just regularly manscape my beastly hairy body because these unintentional waxings keep happening to me.

Another round of questions by the emergency doc on call who gets me admitted. But not before leaving specific written instructions to keep the magnet at my bedside. Even in my depleted state, I insisted on checking his instruction. Amazingly, I could read his doctor scrawl. Or at least I thought I could. Off to the cardiac ward I go. Now I expect that given, you know, the doc wrote specific instructions about keeping the magnet beside me, everything goes smoothly. Silly me. The nurse comes in and says the magnet needs to go back to emergency. You mean to where no one knew what it was for? Absolutely not, I tell her. The doc explicitly wrote that the magnet stays with me. Nurse says it doesn't. I have a screaming match with the nurse, who claims that instruction is not in the chart. Admittedly, it was not one of my better moments, but in my defence, I was exhausted and sick of mistakes being made. I insisted she show me. She gives me the chart and I say "Do I look like a Doris Slobovski (or whatever the name on the chart was) to you? This isn't my chart. Get my chart and don't touch my magnet!" Yep, they sent up the wrong chart with me. As fun as all this had been, the entertainment value was soon to take quantum leaps.

Tangent:

Here comes a quick, state of mind/processing tangent. I'm normally honest. Probably exceedingly honest. So right now, I'm going to up my honesty game. This book has been fucking hard to write. Many will say "Duh! All books are hard to write!" which is 100% true. But I mean ridiculously hard. Likely harder than anything I have done in my life. Obviously challenging, as I had never gone through the process of writing a book before. But I have done a lot of professional writing. There was a lot of learning and acquiring resources along with the writing. But now this is my adventure, so I've learned a few tricks. The first sections had their own challenges, being even more personally traumatic and scientifically or medically more complicated. But this section of the book, yeah. It was beyond a struggle, so even the fact that you are reading it is a miracle.

What made this so crazy? One of the original motives for writing this book was supposed to be therapeutic. Or cathartic. Or rebalancing my perspective. Or hopefully moving off my own cognitive rigidity spots. So yes, it helped with that to a degree. But with this section of the book more than the others, what unexpectedly hit me out of the blue was the absolute rage that leaked out as I wrote. It reinforced how many times the medical community screwed up. Again, this isn't a blame thing. Just what happened for whatever reason. How if I weren't as blessed with smarts as I am (I know, my modesty overwhelms), I wouldn't have been able to advocate for myself and ultimately figure out what was going on. Ultimately, this wouldn't protect me from the Clusterfuck I was once again going to experience. But what a horrible taste in the mouth this leaves behind. And I've done a Ketogenic diet, and if you have also done that, well, you know what an awful taste in the mouth is. And Keto's got nothing on this. Well, you know the old saying "Good things come in threes". Well, I think I am just going to change that to "Good, bad or neutral things come in threes". At least that's my current experience. We'll now return you to the non-state of mind/processing part of the story.

Communication channels in the hospital are always a challenge and probably always will be. Take the following exchange the first morning I was admitted. Me to nurse. Can I get my meds please? Nurse to me - the doctor didn't authorize me to give you any meds. Now let me check your blood sugars. Me – Why check my blood? Her - In case your sugars are high, and you need some insulin. Me, asking incredulously - You mean the insulin you just told me you could not give me? Food was also a continuing issue. This was far from my first time in this hospital. My file definitely has me listed as needing Kosher meals. Of course, the first meal they bring me is… something I would never request - chicken a la king, cream of mushroom soup, milk, and vanilla pudding. To those of you not overly familiar with the Kosher dietary laws, one of the most basic rules is you never mix dairy with meat/poultry. Nothing about this meal was in any way kosher. I remind the orderly who brought the meal, who is the same person who comes around in the morning to take your meal preferences on her tablet. The standard response is "Oh, I have nothing to do with this. Get your nurse to make sure your file is correct". Of course, this isn't true, as she is the one entering the request for the kosher meals on her tablet. Nothing gets changed. Because for my evening snack, I get this: a non-kosher Turkey sandwich, a carton of milk, plus a container of yogurt. It says Kosher Strict right on the label of the yogurt. But nope. We'll get this straightened out. Eventually. If I live long enough. There has to be some fruit around here some place.

AND MY EVENING SNACK - LE SIGH
THE BIG REVEAL AND THE MYSTERY IS
SOLVED!

October 22 - I went through a huge battery of tests, including a few trips to the pacemaker clinic, but wasn't getting much feedback. One day, Dr. Angio comes in and says, "We figured it out. Your pacemaker is malfunctioning". What? How is that possible? How did you figure it out? What happens next? "I'm not the pacemaker expert. I'm just the messenger. I don't have the details. Save your questions for Dr. Kugel". (Kugel, a Yiddish word, is a baked pudding or casserole, most often but not always made from egg noodles. It's obviously not his real name but the name he chose for the book). "Kugel is the pacemaker expert. He and Dr. Pedals should be in this afternoon". Ok, then. No sense in calling people to give them an update because I really had no update to give. I made the mistake of trying to use Dr. Search Engine to look up failed pacemakers and ended up going down a rabbit hole of technical babble. Nothing that gave me any substantive info. At least it helped me kill an hour or so. Eventually, Pedals and Kugel (sounds like an old vaudeville comedy act) arrived. It became clear fairly quickly that Kugel was like Pedals in that they both were direct and to the point.

GETTING A TASTE OF DR. KUGEL

After introducing me to Dr. Kugel, Pedals started off "Well Fred, you presented quite the challenge to us. It was quite the team effort going through all your pacemaker data, determining what is happening, then deciding on a treatment plan." "So doc, don't leave me hanging, what's going on?" Dr. Kugel started in "You either have a cracked pacemaker lead (aka the insulation is cracked) that is preventing the pacemaker signal from firing regularly or there is a malfunction in the lead attachment point doing the same thing. Either way, you need to replace the lead, or this will continue and probably get worse". When are we doing this? "We have to book a slot at Hospital B, so we'll let you know ASAP. Mind if I look at the insertion spot?" Sure, knock yourself out. Which turned out to be the exact wrong phrase to invoke. Kugel presses around the pacemaker and boom, brainquake, fireworks, you know the drill. I come to and Kugel says something like "Jesus Christ, we need to get that out of there ASAP". Just moving the pacemaker triggered the failure. If I moved the wrong way, it failed. Good to know. Pedals and Kugel went off to ensure my ASAP slot was even ASAPer.

ARE YOU THERE, BOTTOM?
HAVE I HIT YOU YET?

Here comes another surgery. I had worked so hard to get my life back. And here I was again, three steps forward, 17 steps back. Truly, I thought I had hit bottom and clawed my way back up and out. Apparently not. I was emotionally deflated. Dear life: if you are going to keep kicking me around like this, at least be fair. If you are going to leave me deflated like this, spread it around. At least deflate my gut as well and leave me six-pack abs. Is that too much to ask? The thought of spending my life in a constant state of continuous pacemaker malfunction and ongoing surgeries isn't a destiny to aspire to.

Even though I get bumped up in the queue, it will still be a few days until the procedure. The days moved slowly. Lots of visitors. A few more stints at the pacemaker clinic. More X-Rays, blood work. The usual. I think. And then something occurs to me. I thought they said all this misfiring was prematurely draining the pacemaker battery. Maybe we could kill two birds with one stone. I wandered over to see Queen Emma, the woman who rules over Pacemakerville and her trusty admin person, Goddess. I really like them. They are great at what they do and super friendly. I asked Emma "If my battery is getting on the lower side and it has to be replaced in a couple of years anyway, wouldn't it make sense to just replace it now during this surgery and save the cost of another operation?" Emma said, "That's a good idea. First, let me see if

Kugel is on board with it and second, let me see if your type of pacemaker is in stock and if they can get it to us on time". Cool. I felt good doing something proactive. Kind of. I guess. Later that day, Kugel came by and said everything was a go – both the new lead and the new pacemaker are available. We'll replace everything and you will be good as new. That definitely boosted my mood and confidence.

Moving day arrives, Wednesday Oct 23, 2013. At 9:00 AM, they ship me off in the transport ambulance. Just to remind you, for the most part, the transport ambulances are regular ambulances that have been run into the ground, sold to a private company, with minor refurbishing. Even minor is a stretch. If you think the ride in a regular ambulance is bad, the transport ambulances are significantly worse. I suspect the horse drawn stagecoaches from 150 years ago had smoother rides. The usual disorientation I experienced from looking out the back window and moving in the opposite direction was amplified in this bucket of bolts. By a wide margin. I'm surprised being bounced around like that didn't short out the pacemaker again. The transport crew wheels me in. I get registered and put in the prep area. I know I must have, but I don't recall going through prep before the first pacemaker surgery in 2009. A Muslim woman, full hijab, comes in to tell me she is going to shave me and douse me with antiseptic. I understand this as "I'm going to shave your chest" as that is where the surgery is going to be, so I start removing my gown. "Underwear too", she adds. Huh? What? "We do your groin area as well in case they have to do any extra insertions". Extra insertions? I don't like the sound of "extra insertions". Yikes. Then I recall they did my first angiogram though the femoral artery that they access through the groin, so it made sense. Little did I know how much of a foreshadowing this would be. She proceeds to clean me up. As she is doing this, I think that this is an odd job for a modest religious woman. Then I realize that often times, we don't get to choose our career path and how we can pay rent/feed out families. I asked how she ended up in this job and she gave me the full refugee experience story. She had no opportunity in her village, got sponsored to move here, got a GED, went to a tech school, then worked her way up to this job. I didn't ask what came before shaving naked men, but good for her, making the most of her opportunities. Hopefully, more would come her way. My surgery was scheduled for 1 PM, but we missed that mark. As per instructions, I had been fasting. Little did I know that this fasting, which seemed torturous to me at the time, would become such an integral part of my life in the future. Around 4 p.m., I said to the nurse that I don't think this is happening today. I should probably eat and have my normal meds. The nurse tried calling the surgical scheduling office (or something like that) and got no response. Finally, she says, "I'll order your meds and find you something to eat. Try not to eat too much as we still want you fasted for whenever you have the surgery". I called Cassie and told her surgery was a no go for today.

I don't know about you, but I find planning for whenever pretty difficult and frustrating. As I am a transfer patient and they weren't expecting to feed me, never mind keep me overnight, so they had no dietary request information filled out. A ham and cheese sandwich, a carton of milk and some yogurt were brought to me. I explained I couldn't eat this as I keep Kosher. She apologized and said this was all that was in the fridge. I teased her and said "Well, your fridge sucks". You know that saying, as one fridge door closes, another fridge door opens? Well, that is exactly what happened. Cassie had called my brother-in-law (we can call him Xylo as in Xylophone). Xylo, along with Xyloette and their little Xylo-munchkins showed up. She didn't tell them to bring me food, but they did. And they brought, oh I'd say, easily food for four people. I thanked them for the food and joked that I'd just had a ham and cheese sandwich with milk and yogurt. The kids were visibly upset seeing me like this, hooked up to wires, monitors beeping with weird displays. I tried to explain how this is a pretty common procedure, what all the technology did, and it was all going to be fine. I showed them how I could make all the displays change by moving around or holding my breath. Not sure if that helped or made it worse. I had a good meal and a better visit. Then, just like that, Xylo and his entourage needed to leave. I wanted him to take the leftovers, but nope, they were for me. The nurse explained the fridge wasn't available to temporary patients. Plus, there was no way to warm the food. In the end, I gave the food to whatever orderlies came by. And suddenly it was the next morning.

Around 6 AM, I was woken for all the usual bloodwork and reading my vitals. A resident came by with the anesthetist to explain what was going to happen. English was definitely not his first language. Maybe Spanish or Portuguese? Possibly South or Central American. Regardless, we understood each other. I thought Dr. Kugel was doing the surgery, but he would just be doing oversight. As long as Kugel was running the show, I was confident things would be ok. Although they really need to get better at telling patients when this doctor flipping is going to happen. It was also the first time I was told I was going to be awake for the procedure. What? You are cutting me open while I'm awake? No worries. We give you a local for the incision site – you won't feel a thing. Well, that promise turned out to be a complete load of crap. Finally, the big moment arrives and another exciting gurney ride, staring at the ceiling and wondering how the ceiling tiles get so dirty. Finally arriving at the lab, I move from the gurney to the operating table. If I thought it was cold in the angiogram lab, it is considerably colder in this lab. I don't recall the first pacemaker lab in 2009 being a freezer like this. I'm taken aback by how many people are involved here. A fair number of nurses, a pacemaker tech (someone from the pacemaker lab) named Georgia, Dr. Kugel and the non-English speaking resident (my apologies if this sounds racist – I am just at a loss for a code name for this doctor). And others I didn't know.

PACEMAKER REPLACEMENT 1.0 – THE CLUSTERFUCK BEGINS

There was a big monitor, almost a scoreboard, that posted my vitals. It allows the doctors to watch where the new lead was going through my veins. Suddenly, a couple of people started wrapping me in a big towel or blanket to pin my arms to my sides. I wasn't aware I was going to be bound up like this. Suddenly, I was feeling quite anxious and claustrophobic, which was a totally new and unpleasant experience for me. I am guessing 50 Shades of Gray is not on my reading list. Then they put this plastic box shield over my head to set up a barrier between me and the incision site, which was on my upper left chest. This made me feel even more anxious. They started dousing me with antiseptics, which put me over the edge. I told them I didn't like this and was having trouble breathing from these fumes. I need this box thing off of me. Then Georgia said they lost signal capture on the big board (the monitor). They tried adjusting the box for better airflow, but it wasn't helping. Dr. non-English told me to try to hold on, we'd be finished before I knew it. And before I knew it, he had numbed the area, then started cutting me with a cauterizing scalpel. The combination of being tied up, smelling my flesh burning, and the antiseptic was overwhelming. And suddenly, I felt a brainquake coming on, then blurted out "Oh fuck, I'm gone". Yep, I could tell before the medical team that my heart had stopped. Before it even showed up on the monitor! I had coded. A full-on code blue. Just a reminder. Code blue indicates a medical emergency, such as cardiac or respiratory arrest. Alas, once again, I was dead.

I don't recall how long I was gone, but the coming back to life was even more brutal than usual. I was extra confused, and someone was pounding on my chest. Like really pounding. You see this on TV or the movies, but this was totally next level. I managed to mutter, "what's going on?" to which some male responded, "Shut up, we are trying to save your life". Then another male yelled, "No, keep talking so we know you are ok!" Glad we are getting the messaging consistent. It was total bedlam. Someone is screaming to get more fucking nurses in here! Another is screaming to get the temporary pacemaker. Whose got it? Where is it? It's in the supply closet. No, it isn't! The pounding and pounding on my chest continues. Ummm, I'm alive again, can whoever keeps pounding my chest please stop? It's really painful. It feels like I'm being repeatedly kicked in the ribs. No one is pounding on you. We're shocking your heart to keep it beating. Now be quiet. No, keep talking, so we know you are good. Where is that fucking pacemaker??? Got it, it's here. Oh, for fuck's sakes, where is the lead? No one said to get the lead! What fucking use is it if we can't connect it? Get a fucking lead!!!! I'll get it. Here, here's the lead. Sterilize it! Ok, we are good to go. Mr. Rutman, this is going to hurt. We have to make an incision in your groin, and we don't have time to sterilize it or freeze it. (Current thought – maybe freeze it and sterilize me while you guys are searching for the temporary pacemaker? Even more current thought – how about while you are sterilizing the lead?) Also, see what I did there? Using "current" while dealing with all this electrical stuff? Yeah, editing is boring. Try not to move. They start cutting. Mother fucker that hurt! Oh my God! The pain is surging through my testicles. Don't move! We want to make sure we get the lead in. Don't move??? You try not moving while someone spears your groin. Threading the lead! Ok, we think it's in. Phew! Finally, the pounding stops. The pain of being sliced open stops, although the getting kicked in the balls pain is still there. Oh my god, that was terrifying, painful, and exhausting. Wow, I feel like shit. Dr. Kugel tells me something but all I remember is "We're taking you back to cardiac ICU and we need to figure out next steps. But try not to move. We have no way of telling how well-anchored that lead is or isn't. We don't want you going through this again". HE doesn't want ME going through this again? I'm damn sure going through this again is NOT on my bucket list.

I believe it was Dr. non-English and a transport porter who wheeled me back to Cardiac ICU. Cassie had arrived and was waiting in my room. To say she was surprised I was back so soon is an understatement. Then Dr. Kugel came in to explain to Cassie what had happened. The post-surgery report (which I only got to see in June 2020) was pretty sparse. Apparently, most of these reports are just a summary of a summary of a summary. This one noted I was only dead for maybe 10 seconds before being revived via the pacing pads. All this chaos was over in 10 minutes. Nothing about the board not capturing my vitals, not having a temporary pacemaker on hand, not being able to find it, not bringing the lead with it, having to go search for that too or not sterilizing and freezing me. I am grateful for the pacing/shocking pads, which are formally called Transcutaneous Pacing, not to be confused with the more familiar defibrillators you see on TV and in the movies. Defibrillators generally deliver one shock, then need to be recharged to deliver a second jolt. Transcutaneous pads are adhesive pads, roughly the size of a slice of toast. One pad stuck to my upper back, the other on my ribs. This allows the current to run between them, through the heart to force it to beat. If memory serves, it fired every ¾ of a second. Of course, I don't recall them placing these on me. Or if they did, I certainly had no idea what they were. Dr. Kugel comes over and apologizes for what happened. He then reiterates that when he says try not to move, he really means try not to move. No getting out of bed to use the washroom, no stretching, no rolling over. Nothing. The temporary lead is in that precarious a position.

The temporary pacemaker will keep me alive until they determine when they can try again. When can they try again? Why can't we just do this again tomorrow? (Hopefully the successful version, not the shit show ride I just went on). Oh, because we weren't able to sterilize the wound site in your groin, you may have gotten an infection. We can't attempt this again until we are sure you have no infection. How long will that take? Maybe up to a week? Are you kidding me? I have to lie here not moving for a week? Sadly yes. Hopefully less, but only the blood work can tell us when. UGH! Kugel leaves and a nurse comes to clean me up a bit. My groin area is a mess, dried blood everywhere. Plus, everything is swollen and hurts like hell. Ah yes, the downside of no freezing. OMG lady, take it easy. It's pretty tender down there. "Oh, I've done this before. I know what I'm doing". "Apparently not", I hiss at her. "They didn't freeze me. Give me the cloth and I'll do it myself!" Apparently, my insisting she not manhandle my super sore testicles offended her. She gave me a "Harrumph!", left the cloth and went away.

I finish cleaning up as best I can. The nurse opens the privacy curtain. Cassie comes to my beside. She doesn't know all the details, but she knows a surgery gone bad. I know I have this temporary pacemaker firing away, but do not know how it works. Because everything else attached to me is plugged into an outlet, I assumed the temporary pacemaker was too. Ok, I hadn't thought it through. How could they keep it plugged in, in the approximately 4-600-meter trip from the pacemaker lab to my room? Obviously you can't. Let's skip over that little inconsistency in my thought process. I put my head back, took an enormous sigh and boom. No, not another brainquake, although that is a damn good guess. Total power outage. Everything went black. And I shit myself because I thought the temporary pacemaker was gone too. But it kept going. Phew. I didn't understand it, but I wasn't complaining. Soon, the generators kicked in, then the main power came back. Please, please, please let the insanity of this day be done with. It wasn't until a few hours later that I learned what was powering the temporary pacemaker. A nurse came by. "Well, we don't know how long this baby was sitting on the shelf, so we'll just swap out the batteries to be safe". Swap out the batteries to be safe? What? It turns out I was being kept alive by a 9-volt battery, sending a charge via a precariously attached lead in my heart. (Battery companies, this is a great product promotion spot. Feel free to contact me and sponsor my podcast). Good lord, a 9-volt battery that was sitting for who knows how long. That wasn't a confidence inspiring moment.

The days of waiting to find out when they could try another surgery were a combination of brutal, boring and being really uncomfortable. At least the swelling and pain in my groin was subsiding. Taking care of the normal bodily functions was the worst. Not being able to shower. Even brushing my teeth lying down was difficult. But the worst was the washroom duties. It wasn't just difficult trying to do things lying flat on a bedpan. Your body just doesn't want to work properly at those angles, especially after it has been traumatized. I mean, even the Squatty Potty tries to get you sitting in a fetus-like position to improve your angles. It turns out that a couple of years later, I became friendly with the Canadian manufacturer of the Squatty Potty, so I am ok giving him the free plug. Layer all the trauma my body just went through, and it adds up to a world class case of constipation. I had forgotten about this bonus from the first surgery in 2009. People forget that nurses have to deal with things like this as a part of patient care. I'm sure enemas and cleaning up after bowel movements isn't on the front of the "So you are considering a career in nursing?" promotional brochures. Obviously, some nurses are better at dealing with issues like this than others. This really is a well-known post-surgery phenomenon. It's puzzling why they don't start pumping you with fibre as soon as possible. Or even before the surgery. Thankfully, after about three days, one nurse took me seriously and took the appropriate action. What a relief. Literally. A huge relief.

NURSE RATCHED 2.0

Just like any occupation, there is a wide range of quality/skill level in the nursing profession. All the ICU nurses were top notch. Ok, just like my 2009 ICU experience, there was one exception – the unforgettable Nurse Ratched. It wasn't that the care this new nurse provided me was substandard. It was just that she was a bitter person. Beyond bitter, in fact. She was a racist. She was constantly complaining about how all her neighbours were immigrants, were taking all the jobs, and never came over to say hello or introduce themselves. I asked how long she had been in her home. She said 20 years. She moved in after her divorce. After probably her 10th time telling me this "story", I made the mistake of saying something like "Well, I am not an expert on this but usually it is the long-time resident who welcomes the newcomers to the neighbourhood". She didn't like this pearl of wisdom at all. She knew how uncomfortable and anxious I was to get my surgery retry. Rachet 2.0 soon returned to inform me she had checked the schedule and it was booked solid. Really solid. I would be lucky if I got cleared for surgery in the next two weeks, if not longer. I was less than thrilled hearing this. And at shift change, the next nurse told me this was BS. They don't even have access to the schedule, and I was top priority. Nurse Racist Ratched was just lashing out at me. She's just not a happy person. Fortunately, I was released before she came back on rotation.

As you might expect, waiting for the days to pass was pretty boring when all you can do is lay in bed motionless. Cassie tried playing some board and card games with me but it's really difficult to do that when you aren't able to see the board. She knows I can't visualize things like that, so I think it was all part of her secret plan to keep me from winning any games. Ah, good times staring at the ceiling. At the other hospital and in the previous hospital, I had access to patient lounges so a fair number of people could visit at once. Here, I was strapped to the bed, so this capped me at one or two people per visit. Overall, the title of most visits was a tie between Mr. Jeans 2.0 and Mr. Borsalino (he almost always wears a formal black hat). I kept a log of all my visitors and Sunday's tally was 62 people. I remember the total but lost my journal somewhere. Even friends who have a really hard time dealing with hospitals showed up. It looked like my buddy Calcutta (his birth city) was going to toss his cookies. But he didn't. Speaking of cookies, his wife makes amazing cookies (I sampled some last week, August 2020). Truly, she is an amazing cook and baker. As a side note (August 2022), Calcutta and I went for a walk. That hospital visit, and how difficult it is for him to be in a hospital, came up. I told him how much I appreciated him doing that. During the pandemic, a small group of us sometimes get together at Calcutta Manor on Sabbath afternoons. They have a big enough front patio that allows visiting while socially distanced. And Mrs. Calcutta never disappoints. Last week was blueberry flange – absolutely amazing. Plus, a huge shout out to the Calcuttas for Beta reading my manuscript.

PACEMAKER REPLACEMENT 2.0 –
THE CLUSTERFUCK CONTINUES

Sunday was a crazy, exhausting day with the 62 visitors. The nurses told me they had never seen anything like it – a constant parade of people to see me. To quote Sally Field "They like me. They really, really like me!" It wasn't quite a full week since the first surgery debacle. So far, my bloodwork was showing no infection, so they scheduled me for attempt number two Monday morning. Yay! The end is in sight. Freedom is around the corner. Cassie had to return home for family and work reasons. Thank God she had come for the time she did. In no way did I want a repeat of surgery number one, so I asked to see the surgeon and anesthetist before the procedure. I was told Dr. Kugel wasn't available so it would be a doctor from this hospital and – wait for it – Dr. non-English again. Seriously, hadn't I suffered enough? But I had no say in the matter. Ok, what did I want to chat about? Obviously, I was hooked up to the temporary pacemaker already, so I was protected against my heart stopping again mid-procedure. That is, as long as they remembered to change the batteries. So that left the claustrophobia from being tied up and the plastic box over my head, the fumes from the antiseptic and the burning flesh from the cauterizing scalpel to deal with. Dr. non-English comes by and tries to push off my concerns, which pissed me off to no end. Finally, I said (and this was aggressive, even for me), "Seeing as though it seems no one has told you, instilling confidence in your patients is a big part of your job. Telling me to chill is not an appropriate response from you. The response I'm looking for is, "I will talk it over with the team and we'll figure this out. You find a way to deal with this shit or I'm going to find a way to get you booted off the team. And I want to know what we are going to do before the procedure starts". Damn, these surgeons can uniquely combine obliviousness and arrogance. What kind of surgeon wants his patient having a panic attack mid-procedure? Not a good one, that's for sure. If only my friend MacGreaveser were here. She'd rig up a fix in three minutes. Guaranteed.

Keeping the timeline straight, it's now Monday, October 28, 2013. I'm first in line for the pacemaker lab. Georgia the pacemaker tech is one of my escorts for this gurney ride. She half giggles/half tells me Dr. non-English shared my concerns and that I kind of rattled him with how aggressive I was. Good, at least I got him to take some action beyond telling me to chill. So what changes are we going to make? Georgia listed them off: "We are going to use a traditional scalpel, instead of the cauterizing scalpel, so no fumes. We are using a different antiseptic that shouldn't affect you as much. We've added a fan to the box to keep the fumes away from you, plus we are going to give you a little anti-asthma and anti-anxiety medicine before we start". Fan-freaking-tastic. Just hearing this calmed me down. All should go swimmingly. Right? (Note, this is called foreshadowing. It won't go swimmingly. Whatever swimmingly means). We arrive in the lab, which is still super cold. I meet the new head Doctor. Dr. Kugel had called me and told me this guy was top notch, so I was in excellent hands. They go through all the prep, and all seems in order. Minimal fumes, minimal anxiety. We're good to go. The freezing is injected and in 45 minutes, I'll be back in the Cardiac ICU. And soon after that, I'll also be able to move. Again, more foreshadowing.

Everything started off well. All the accommodations seemed to be holding up. The freezing goes in. The incision was made. If I remember the order of things correctly, the first order of business was to disconnect the original pacemaker's leads so that the original pacemaker could be removed. The temporary pacemaker leads are the last to go. I didn't realize, nor did anyone mention, that this is not a simple task. Dr. non-English pulled out some sort of Hex Key device to loosen things up. He really had to crank to detach the leads. I was surprised at the amount of torque required. Task one completed. The temporary pacemaker is running smoothly. Task two begins: threading the new lead in. Remember, I am fully awake through all this. Or at least I started off awake. I really don't know if I simply fell asleep from exhaustion. Maybe I passed out. Or worse. I do know I kept waking up and finding new Head Doctor either on the phone or on a video chat. And no one was working on me. At one point, I woke up and asked, "What's going on?" I received the stern response, "Be quiet. We are trying to figure out how to fix your situation". My situation? What situation? You were supposed to fix my existing situation, not create an additional one. What the fuck is happening now? Zzzzzzz. Two or three times, I woke up in significant pain and had to ask for more freezing. Which, surprisingly, they had on hand. Then I woke up and there was a third surgeon in the room. Third surgeon and new Head Doctor were on a video chat with whom knows who, discussing who knows what. But I wasn't being worked on. I looked at the clock. It was well past 2 hours. Well, I got bumped last week. Unfortunately, I guess someone else is getting bumped out of their surgery slot this week. It sucked for me. Sorry it will suck for them. Finally, I wake up and they are working on me again. Somehow, they rectified whatever issue they had. I won't find out about what the issue was until about two years later while getting another medical issue checked out. It's now time to put in the new pacemaker and reattach the leads. And ummm, can you guess what happens next? They ordered a different sized pacemaker, which was too big for the existing "pocket". The pocket is the space opened up under your skin and above the muscle for the pacemaker to reside in. Seriously guys? As they say in every episode of the TV show MacGyver (the reboot, not the original), "Mac, what are we going to do?" "Improvise!" Normally, I like improvisation. In fact, I used to take improv classes. It seems both procedures were one continuous improvisation. I couldn't see if non-English grabbed an instrument or just dug his hand in like a jackhammer – dig, dig, dig, slam, slam, slam–pealing the tissue off the muscle to make more space. Even though I was frozen, I could still feel this. If I wasn't going to be bruised like hell tomorrow from the previous surgery attempt, I sure am now. A couple more attempts and the new pocket was ready to accept the pacemaker. Just a simple attaching of the leads – crank, crank, crank – detaching the temporary pacemaker, 20 or so stitches to the chest and groin and we are done. Three and a half hours later. The most convoluted pacemaker/lead replacement in history was complete. Here's a hint for later: remember that the post-surgery reports are just a summary of a summary of a summary. None of these difficulties were detailed in the report.

They keep me in Cardiac ICU for a couple more days and finally I get released. The last order of hospital business is to weigh me. I do not know why. If the scales here are accurate, I've lost 16 lbs in 9 days on the new and improved Defective Pacemaker Diet. #FindingLittlePositives #TrademarkPending The release, of course, is predicated on my having someone to escort me home. You can't just order a ride share or taxi and disappear. I am fortunate that even though I have no family in Toronto, I have many friends who treat me like family. One of those families is the Jeans. I already mentioned Mr. Jeans 2.0. This is about Mr. Jeans 1.0, the older brother. Mrs. Jeans 1.0 arranged for Mr. Jeans 1.0 to pick me up and get me home. Now I had known them for a number of years but had never driven with them. Mr. Jeans 1.0

does everything fast. I mean really fast. Walks fast, talks fast, eats fast, thinks fast. And now I learned he drives fast. Really fast! One of the many things I've learned on this journey is that people don't get the concept of surgery. Even if they have had surgery themselves. By that I mean they know you had a surgery to fix/treat whatever. That part is obvious. What they don't get is that even though you are being released from the hospital, you are nowhere close to healed and are still pretty fragile. Which I was. In fact, I was told no driving (that is, no me being the driver) or public transport for 10 weeks! I had to either be chauffeured or take a cab everywhere. I also wasn't allowed to travel/fly. This fragility, when combined with someone's fast aggressive driving, was a less than pleasant experience. The abrupt changing lanes, the late braking, the sudden accelerations, the hard cornering just throws you all over the car. Which is exactly what you don't need at that point. Although it was not as overtly stupid as after my 2009 surgery, when some clown at synagogue came up behind me and slapped me on the back, "Hey, I heard you just had heart surgery!" He was a big guy so when I say slap, I mean knocked the wind out of me and I fell into the pews. Anyhow, Jeans 1.0 eventually got me home with a couple of new bruises, and I went right to sleep for about 6 hours. Home, where I can shower and once again pee upright. Although not at the same time. Let the healing begin. (Hint: this is more foreshadowing).

It's Halloween eve, one of my favourite holidays. I wish there were more kids wandering into our little cul-de-sac. There are two reasons for this: One, seeing little kids all dressed up and excited is fun; Two, there would be way less junk left for me to eat. The last couple of years, I even started putting my super bright bike light in the window, set on flashing mode, to attract some kids wandering down the main road. It got a few newbies, but nothing significant. Unfortunately, in my current state, handing out candy for an hour was all I could handle. I was exhausted and needed a nap. Or three. I guess this is what newborns feel like.

The next day, I wanted to get a walk in before Shabbat starts. I want to gauge if I might be able to walk to Synagogue Saturday morning. Except I encounter a bit of a stumbling block – I can't get my apartment door open. I come in through the backdoor of the house. My fabulous friends decided independently they were all going to make me meals for the weekend. Except they didn't tell me this and all piled the food outside my door, essentially locking me in. There was probably enough food for 10 days! I called my elderly neighbour Spielberg (he was in the movie biz) to come excavate me, which he was more than happy to do. He was also an ex-Winnipegger who knew a couple of my late uncles from their high school sports days. After he extricated me, I grabbed a couple of adult beverages (which neither of us probably should have had). We sat out on the deck. Even after all these years, I still enjoy hearing tales of days gone by in the Peg. Unfortunately, with me moving from the neighbourhood and my subsequent medical adventures, Mr. Spielberg and I lost touch. No one told me he passed away, so I missed his funeral. A few times I've been back to the old neighbourhood. I've knocked on the door a couple of times to see Mrs. Spielberg but so far, we haven't connected.

After our visit, I ended up walking about two thirds of the way to synagogue and back, which seemed about my limit. Then Mama Borsalino called to invite me for Sabbath lunch. Perfect. I could walk to the synagogue, then chill at their place. They would drive me home after Sabbath ends. Spending time with the Borsalinos and their clan is always a good time. In fact, it was such a good time that I also spent the entire next weekend with them. Because on Wednesday, November 6, my brand new, barely out of the box pacemaker glitched again. Another brainquake, smacking my head and coming back to life with a crazy fireworks display. This can't be happening again, can it?

Another day, another ambulance ride. Yes, I am back in Hospital B for a few days (hopefully no more). Might be a glitch in the new pacemaker so they are keeping an eye on me. You could not plan a more fun vacay. Cabo San Pacemaker. It's number one on most travel sites. Seriously, this isn't the type of staycation I should be taking. The first 18 hours were in emergency. I was hooked up to the monitors and the readings were crazy. My heart rate was at a constant 175 beats per minute. But it wasn't. I wasn't breathing hard nor was I out of breath. I didn't feel my heart pounding. To be honest, haven't really been able to feel my heart pounding since the first pacemaker implant in 2009. It really has to be pumping hard for me to notice it. Not sure what they did to me or if this is a normal outcome from having a pacemaker. I'm generally on the continuum of breathing normally, breathing hard or being out of breath. But I rarely have heart sensation. I was sweating and my blood pressure was on the higher side. Aside from that, I had no symptoms beyond the big syncope. I was quite anxious. Freaking out level anxious. I've never experienced anything like this. Eventually, I fell asleep. Then finally a doctor came in. And by finally, I mean at some point Thursday morning. Apparently, there were no cardiologists available to come to emergency all night, which I found kind of mind boggling. We can call him Dr. Clooney – He had that suave movie star look. He was a foreign doctor on a fellowship to learn some sub or sub-sub-specialty of heart treatment. He starts off with something like – this isn't my area of expertise, but hey, I have some free time, so I thought I'd see what was going on. So basically he drew the newbie short straw. And we just chatted. Turns out he was renting a place about five blocks from where I live – and from people I know. He agreed that something was off – he was thinking the monitor, not the pacemaker. Although that wouldn't explain the syncope and bump on my head. Dr. Clooney said he wants me admitted and he is personally going to go through every piece of data from my pacemaker log. He added that when we figured things out and if I was up to it, we could go for a bike ride together. That calmed me down a lot. Sadly, he went back to his home country before we could get a ride in.

Somehow, some people found out I was back in the hospital and started coming to visit. I likely called someone or posted it on social media. One of the local Rebbetzins (The title for a Rabbi's wife) popped in. They are known in the neighbourhood as Momma and Daddy Spider, names given to them by a member of a local group home resident they befriended. The Spiders are another one of the amazing families in my community. I've lost count of how many times I have been to their home for meals and great conversation. "I'm so sorry, I can't stay long. We are going to a wedding out of town. I didn't have time to cook so the best I could do is bring you store bought". And she presented me with two shopping bags of munchies. I thought it was amazing that she came to see me at all. All she had on her schedule was to pack and wrangle her seven kids and her hubby, then get them to the airport and through customs. No time constraints there. And yet she found time to make the trip to the store, to the hospital, visit me for half an hour, then scoot back home and get to the airport.

Hanna Solo also dropped by. With a couple of slices of pizza, of course. Outside of my hospital adventures, maybe once a month, Hanna also offers me "leftovers". She and her hubby host a lot of guests for Sabbath (when there is no Covid Pandemic Lockdown), so there are lots of leftovers. This week, August 2020, Hanna messaged me to come get some barbequed meatloaf goulash. No guests obviously. She just made too much. And yes, it was amazing. A couple of hours after the visitors, they are shipping me up to the cardiac ward. On the way, I see Dr. Clooney working away on my pacemaker report. It looked like literally hundreds of mind-numbing pages of heart signals, even though I've only had this pacemaker for a week. Yep, your heart beats that much. I appreciate him making the effort.

ENTER THE MISSIONARIES

We get to my room and the nurse comes in. "Where do you want me to post these?" "Post what?" "Your inspirational material". "I have my own inspirational material and people thanks". "Oh no, sir. You have nothing like this". And she starts putting up pictures of Jesus and sayings from the New Testament. I'm mildly offended, but it's not worth my energy to deal with her. Although, for the charge nurse, that is a different story. She definitely had the energy. "Debbie!!!" she screamed (not the nurse's real name). "Dammit, we've talked about this. You aren't allowed to evangelize with patients. Now take it all down. This is your last warning before I officially reprimand you". Well, I didn't see that coming. Awkward. Then the guy in the bed next to me started yelling at the charge nurse, "Leave her alone. She can practice freedom of religion. This is a free country!" "Freedom of religion is for your personal practices. It doesn't allow you to impose your beliefs in the workplace and on patients who don't ask for it". This went back and forth for a few minutes. Finally, I just blurted out, "All of you shut up. This is ridiculous. I'm in here because I've been really sick and want to get better. Your behaviour in here isn't helping me in any way. I politely told you I don't want your propaganda. You ignored me. Get rid of it now and stay out of my room. And you Sir (I stared at the guy in the bed like I've never stared at anyone before), I don't want to hear one word from you.

About anything. Got it?" And that was that. Shortly after, the very smart charge nurse had my roomie put in another room. Not surprisingly, while I was napping, Debbie snuck in and put up more JC material. Dr. Clooney came by, said he found the syncope event, but no idea why it happened. Could be I simply moved the wrong way? This was news to me. I thought this new pacemaker was supposed to prevent that kind of thing from happening. He said he was going to keep me over night again, run more tests and see if there is something more obvious. Then he suggested we do a couple of laps around the ward so he can watch me and see if something shows up. Sounds good to me. I start to get out of bed, stand up and boom, brainquake and I'm out cold. Thankfully, Dr. Clooney was able to partially grab me, preventing another head shot. Well, if he wanted something more obvious, he certainly got it. Clooney may be movie star handsome, but he's no Mr. Olympia. A few people were needed to help me back into bed. When I was finally back and alert, Dr. Clooney said he was fairly sure he knew what was going on – it wasn't the pacemaker messing up. It was my body.

Dr. C's theory is that my venous system was confused due to all the trauma it's endured. Basically, my blood pressure control system (there is that vagus nerve again) was now out of whack. If I got up too quickly (or what my body now decided was too quickly) or moved a certain way, my blood pressure wasn't staying constant, and I would pass out. He was going to get some Physio or Occupational therapists in to work with me on mitigating these situations. For now, rest. We'll run a couple more tests and enjoy your visitors. Visitors? What visitors? I forgot my friend SWT was having an eye procedure at the hospital. She had messaged me she and Dr. Fun (her hubby) would come by after her procedure. Great, although having had a couple of eye procedures myself, I suspected it would be a quick visit. We had a nice visit, and, of course, in the middle of it, an orderly came and says I need to go for a test. I get into the wheelchair with no incident, and then a second orderly joins us. I'm back on fall alert status, so I get two very big manly men to make sure I stay upright. As I am rolling away, I see two more visitors, Mrs. Jeans 2.0, and Mrs. Invisalign. I ask my escorts to hang a second so I can say hi and tell them that there are other visitors in the room. So if you can, just wait with them. Off we rolled. I think it was just a simple chest X-ray to make sure nothing had displaced, but the wait time was pretty long. When I finally got back to the room, there were no visitors. But they left me a note that they brought food for me and left it at the nursing station. The ladies were concerned I might get stuck in the hospital again over the Sabbath, so they stocked me up. Which I appreciated. Off I went to the nursing station. "Hi. I understand my friends left some food for me". The nurse responded that the food wasn't compliant with a diabetic diet, so she didn't want me eating it. That lead to another conversation that only seems to happen to me. "Why would you think it's not compliant?" "Most people don't know how to make a diabetic compliant meal". "My friends cook for a social service agency that is strict with their dietetics. They know I'm diabetic. This is fine". "I can't take your word for it". "Will you take Dr. Clooney's word for it? He's familiar with the agency". "He's not even from here. How would he know the agency, and how would you know he knows it?" "He's an Orthodox Jew. Every Orthodox Jew knows about this service. Just ask him". "That seems unlikely. I'm not paging him for this". "Suit yourself. The organization has a drop off point in the hospital. Which means it is hospital approved. And approved by the orthodox doctors who work here". At this point, the charge nurse comes by "What are you two chatting about?" "We are chatting about why this drop off food is not appropriate for Fred to eat". "Oh, why is that?" "I'm concerned it's not a diabetic compliant meal". "I explained that Dr. Clooney would approve this". "As would I, but that's a different issue". The nurse asked, "What is the issue?" "The issue is, Fred is not your patient, so you shouldn't be making this call". Oh oh. This was a turn I wasn't expecting. I didn't want to be anywhere near this throwdown, so I decided this would be a good time to head back to my room. I wish I were better at not only recognizing these no-win conversations, never mind getting drawn into them. Through a lot of effort, the June 2021 version of me is much better at this.

A few more visitors and a CT scan later, my day was done. My daytime nurse was truly spectacular. I'll call her Resi, as in resilient. It seemed I was her only patient, just like being in ICU – having one nurse assigned to you and only you. I never got the full story, but Resi seemed to be fighting through or recovering from some neurological disorder that impaired her movement. She never complained and had an amazing attitude. And I say this with full respect as she has obviously gone through a lot. If you ever saw Tim Conway's old man characters on the Carol Burnett show, Resi could play his female counterpart. Find a video online. Although my favourite Tim sketch is not one of his old man sketches. It is a tie between The Dentist and the Siamese elephants. Friday morning rolls around. Dr. Clooney says he is not seeing anything to keep me around, pending my time with the OT/PT going well. The therapist drills me on the seven-count stand up, the five-count sit down, the full body turnaround (instead of just turning my head to look at something), and the no-lean over bend to pick things up (bend those knees!). After about 45 minutes of this and no signs of a syncope, the therapist says if it is ok with Dr. Clooney, I am good to go. It takes a while to track down Dr. Clooney. He arranges my discharge papers - I am soon to be free! Of course, I just can't call a ride share. I have to find someone to escort me home. I put the call out on social media to see who might be around.

To my surprise, Mama Borsalino said she'd come and pick me up. I was surprised because the Borsalinos often have guests for Sabbath dinner and at this time of year, sundown, which starts the Sabbath, was about 5 PM. This didn't leave much time to get everything ready for the guests, never mind coming to pick me up, get me home and get herself home. Now I have to pack up my go bag, get my discharge papers and literally ride off into the sunset with Mama B. (Insert movie background music setting the mood for frantic action). I wander to the nursing station to get my discharge papers. The conversation went something like this: "Last I saw, Nurse Resi has your papers. Oh, where is Resi? We think she went to the cafeteria for a break. She'll probably be back in 20 or 30 minutes? Wait, what? Why would she take my papers with her? That makes no sense. I need my papers. I need to get home before sundown". "Sorry pal, we all need something, right?" Arrrrgh! I wonder if this is payback for the two nurses getting in trouble. The clock is ticking, the sun is setting, Mama B arrives, and we are stuck until Resi shows up. We are both getting antsy. Driving on the Sabbath is a big no-no for us. Resi finally returns. "Your papers are right here. Anyone could have given them to you". Then I realize the nurse who wasn't helpful was Debbie, the one who was putting up the JC posters in my room and got in trouble. Hey lady, you got in trouble on your own – I had nothing to do with you not being able to take orders from your boss. Don't take your problems out on me! Papers in hand, I return to my room to get my go bag. "Not so fast," Resi calls out. "You're not quite done. I need to take out your IV and blood catheters (the needle/tube things)". You can try to explain Resi's challenges to someone, but you really need to experience it to appreciate that she is still a highly functional nurse. Mama B called home and warned them she was going to be right on the bubble time-wise. Resi started peeling the tape off me. I really urge you to watch one of the Old Man clips at this point. It was like watching life in super-slow motion. Mama B explained to Resi our urgency to get going for Sabbath and asked if she could go faster. Resi turned to her, and deadpan responded, "Sorry, this IS me going faster. It's the best I can do". It was pretty funny. Of course, it all worked out. Resi got the catheters out, bandaged me up and off we went. As we drove, Mama B said there was no way she could get me home and then get home on time herself, so I was staying at their place for Sabbath. That was fine by me. Cassie called as we were heading to Borsalino manor, so I put her on speaker. Cassie and Mama B knew about each other but had never met or talked, so this would be their first experience with each other. With everything going on, I forgot about the legend of Mama B; That she can sometimes get a biiiiit distracted while driving. As Mama B and Cassie are chatting, I suddenly realize we are now going the wrong way on a one-way street! I grab the phone back, get us out of the traffic death spiral and headed home again. What is it with people driving me home from the hospital trying to put me back in the hospital???

Things sort of normalized, you know, in a Fred kind of way. Dad's 85th birthday was coming up, and we were going to have a big party. His older sisters were 87 and 89. I asked an actuary friend what the odds were of three siblings, all surviving past the age of 85. He did a rough calculation and said maybe 1 in 10,000. Pretty amazing. Alas, I wasn't allowed to fly. They postponed the party until January when my travel ban was lifted. I started exercising and tried taking some additional social media courses to judge if I might be getting ready to return to the corporate world. I noticed this post on my FB feed: November 12, 2013 - Walk #1 is in the books. One mile in 37 minutes #UsainBoltGotNothingOnMe. I mean, it was so slow people could barely tell I was moving. Now I can easily do a mile in 18 minutes. Not great but getting there. Physically, I was feeling ok but far from 100%. I still had depth perception, balance, memory, and speech issues. One thing that really bothered me was that now the weather was colder, my hands were literally freezing. Even indoors. Now Toronto cold is nothing compared to Winnipeg cold, so this was really unsettling. A Winnipegger's ability to tolerate cold is kind of a badge of honour, so this hurt. In fact, it was slightly embarrassing. I mean, I grew up playing hockey outside in -30 Celsius weather without blinking. And that was before factoring in the wind chill. I bought progressively more and more expensive gloves. No help at all. I switched to mitts. Never in my wildest dreams did I think I'd go from the decades old Winnipeg staple $12 Orange "Garbage Mitts" to $230 Alpine mitts. It's a good thing Mountain Equipment Co-op has a liberal return/exchange program. The mitts helped but not completely. I had to also fill them with those ski warmer packets and even those were minimally effective. It was even worse when I went back to the actual cold of Winnipeg. I couldn't even take my mitts off to insert a loonie to access a shopping cart. I'd have to rely on the kindness of strangers. But I got to go home, see family and friends. Plus have a great celebration for my parents. My mom's birthday was in January 2014, so we just did a double birthday party. Actually, it turned out to be a triple as it was also my cousin's mother-in-law's birthday. Sadly, it was the last time I saw my aunts and my dad together. Dad passed in June 2015. But not before giving me one more gift. That gift being a serious case of adult onset chicken pox.

SOMETIMES IT'S ALL IN VEIN

Back to my freezing hands. Dr. Coif arranged to send me to a vascular surgeon, Dr. Vein. He was actually the second vascular surgeon I had seen. The first one was a guy in my neighbourhood who had been referred by a friend. And I didn't even have to shlep to his office! Just went to the house a few blocks from my house. He looked me over, did some manipulations and said he would send me for some follow-up tests, but yeah, something wasn't right with my hands. Oh, sure, he took my health insurance info, Dr. Coif's info, etc. Except we never heard from him again. Dr. Coif found out why we were ghosted but never shared it with me, so on to Dr. Vein. I heard the first doctor (not Dr. Vein) was disbarred or whatever it is they do to doctors when they tell them they can't be doctors anymore. I had a couple of great visits with Dr. Vein. He was a real fashion/suit guy. I even learned a lot about buying suits in Asia, where you can get a custom suit in three days for few hundred dollars or less. Well, except for the $1000s you spend on airfare, food, hotels, being a tourist, etc. Unless you are going to a medical conference. Then you get to write off travel expenses. He said one of his best scores was on Savile Row in London. That's where many of the super high-end bespoke tailors have hung their shingles for more than a few decades. If you are super lucky, you find a shop that has a suit someone never picked up, is in your size that and is still in style. Chances are good as classic suits have long style lives. Much of it was already paid for by the person who never picked it up, so you can get it for a song. If that kind of thing suits you (see what I did there?).

Dr. Vein sent me for a Doppler scan – basically an ultrasound investigation and mapping of my arteries and veins. I love talking to the techs and hearing their stories. The Doppler tech was actually a Radiologist in his homeland, who obviously thought coming to Canada would be better for his family. He decided he didn't think going back to school for 10 years or however long to get his Canadian doctor credentials instead of earning a living was in his best interest. He already had the Doppler skills from his Radiology training, had to do minimal studying, didn't have to go into debt and got his Doppler Technician credential very quickly. And now two of his kids are in med school here. A relatively good ending. I hear stories like this all the time. I remember meeting a gentleman working a hot dog cart. He said he was a nuclear engineer. Ran a major nuclear power plant somewhere in the Former Soviet Union but here, no one recognizes his degrees or credentials. There must be a better system for keeping these skilled immigrants contributing at their same or near-same levels. A couple of weeks later at the follow up with Dr. Vein, he asked me if I knew the vein that they threaded the pacemaker lead through had totally collapsed. Nope, that was news to me. And just a tad disturbing. Veins and arteries expand and contract to control your blood pressure. This vein was now stuck in severe contraction mode. Likely forever. Basically, this means the vein is now so tight around the pacemaker leads that no blood can pass through it. And the light bulb goes off!!! This explains why they couldn't access it during the Pacemaker Replacement Attempt 2.0 – The Clusterfuck Continues surgery. And possibly why the insulation cracked and shorted me out. The vein must have been collapsed right after or during a prior surgery as a response to trauma. It likely wasn't collapsed during the aborted first Clusterfuck surgery because they got nowhere near that far into the procedure.

Which only leaves the original pacemaker surgery in July 2009. Then I remembered I didn't recall having the anaesthesia mask on and no one telling me they were about to put me to sleep. Altogether, this makes me wonder if something happened during my surgery. And as I write this (June 2021), if the doctors from Clusterfuck 2.0 knew this was an issue, shouldn't they have set up some sort of "Be on the lookout" or monitoring system? It seems obvious to me something prophylactic should have been initiated.

A QUICK TRIP BACK TO AREA 51

Again, this is just a theory – but seeing as nothing else had gone right in this (mis)adventure, I think I am pretty justified going down this path. The premise is that I wasn't put to sleep, but that I coded (aka my heart stopped yet again) on the table and the surgery changed from a normal pacemaker implant to an emergency implant procedure. Worldwide, they do 750,000 plus pacemaker surgeries a year (probably more by now) and have been doing them for decades. Meaning they have it down to a science and try to make it as low a trauma as possible, even though each procedure has its own personality. In an emergency procedure, they probably would have had to get a bit rough while expediting the insertion of the pacemaker leads, inflicting trauma on the vein resulting in its collapse. Our bodies, being the miraculous machines they are, will adapt over a couple of months and find alternate routes to deliver the blood. There is no actual damage. You know, beyond the contraction being so severe that it likely damaged the leads and is perpetually trying to kill me. It's just another sign that something went wrong. And no one said boo.

If this is really what happened in the operating room, it definitely clarifies a few things for me:

Why I don't recall being put under,

Why the nurse said I scared the shit out of them, and

Why I felt so horrifically bad after the surgery, which is now fairly routine and low trauma.

I also don't recall the surgeon or anesthetist checking on me after the surgery. Well, the surgeon makes sense, as he was probably running straight to the airport. I've run into elderly men (well into their 80s) in the neighbourhood who just had pacemakers implanted and they seemed a lot less damaged than I was. I was getting a haircut when one of these elderly guys came in on the way home from the hospital, perky as, well, whatever things are really perky. I know the gentleman's grandson and Gramps is in his mid-80s. This was certainly vastly different from my experience. Despite Dr. Vein's diligence, he could not determine what was going on with my hands. We classed it as one of those things that your body will resolve when it decides to resolve it. In the meantime, consider getting some gloves with battery operated heaters. Unfortunately, at $600 or so, they were just a tad beyond my budget. Unless, of course, some electric glove manufacturer wants to do some product placement here or podcast deal. Hey, if you never ask...

THE INTRODUCTION OF
THE VENTRICLE WHISPERER

Time keeps going and I am just seeing Dr. Pedals for my normal four-month check-up (October 2016). I get my ultrasound done, see the doc and all seems well. Yay me! About a week later, I get a call from Pedal's assistant. Dr. P thinks he might see something in your echo, so he wants you to go for a couple of tests outside the office. It looks like you might have a thickening of the ventricle wall. One is for a Nuclear Imaging Test and the second is an appointment with the Ventricle Whisperer. Good grief. It never entered my mind that I would have any other heart issues. The wonky electrical was more than enough for me. On the upside, the wall thickening wasn't so overt that you could tell definitively. How bad could it be? Of course, I started searching Dr. Search Engine to find out why this was a problem. I really need to end my relationship with Dr. Search Engine. It seems that the thicker your walls, the harder it is for your heart to pump. Well, duh, I should have clued into that. Great. Just great. I have to get the nuclear imaging done before I can see the Ventricle Whisperer. The imaging is about a 12-hour fast, followed by a four-hour adventure, in which you down a few shots of radioactive material, wait until it gets absorbed in your system, then sit in a chair that takes film of the radiation working its way through your heart. Fun stuff. Doesn't make you nauseated at all. Ok, maybe a little.

Or maybe a fair bit. Ok, I wasn't the only one running to the washroom. The most fascinating part of all this was the waiting room, where I was sitting across from a guy wearing the worst hairpiece of all time. Dad and his colleagues went through the hairpiece phase back in the day, so I know horrible hair pieces. This guy was surely on the Mount Rushmore of bad rugs. What made him truly epic was that he doubled down with a 1970's Pornstache. It was just mesmerizing.

With that adventure in the books, a few weeks went by. Now it was time to meet the Ventricle Specialist, aka the Ventricle Whisperer. Waiting in the exam room, I hear the click-click-click of stilettos coming down the hall. I'm not positive, but I might have heard angels singing. In comes the Ventricle Whisperer. She was already close to six feet tall and still went for the heels. In my opinion, she could easily be a Victoria's Secret angel, assuming VS Angels still exist. Very stylishly dressed. After we chatted a bit, I half asked, half teased, "I need to know. Are your shoes Louboutin's?" For those of you who don't know, Christian Louboutin is a very high-end fashion line. Shoes can easily be $800 a pair or more. She replied, "I don't know, what's a Louboutin?" I said "Are you kidding me? Seriously, you don't know? It's a high-end fashion line". The Ventricle Whisperer replied, "Sorry, I don't do the high-end stuff. I got these shoes for maybe $22 at a discount mall in Calgary!" We chatted a bit more, then went to find her assistant to set up a couple more tests for me. See you in a month or so, Doc. In the interim, I do a special type of treadmill stress test and some blood work for genetic markers related to ventricle issues. I guess in the good old days, these marker tests came back fairly quickly. Now, everyone wants genetic info on everything. It appears the lab capacities haven't kept up. It took a year to get my test results, which thankfully showed no predisposition to having thickened ventricle walls. I got the nuclear imaging and stress test results back relatively quickly. The Ventricle Whisperer said as there were no abnormalities, there was no need for a follow up. Then she added, "But keep an eye on those ejection fraction numbers". My what? Ejection what? She explained that ejection fraction is the amount of blood pumped out of the ventricle versus the total amount of blood in the ventricle at the time of the pump, expressed as a percentage. Got it? Good. Ideally, you want your ejection fractions over 60%. Under 40% is becoming problematic. Mine was in the mid-40s. Subsequently, Pedals and my cardiologist friend both told me not to worry about the numbers. They both had patients with fractions in the 20s that were perfectly fine. Everyone's body works differently. And except for my electrical issues, I seemed to get enough oxygen despite my lower number. So, all is good, right? Riiiight.

Can I go on a bit of a tangent again? So here was my Pandora's Box, aka the super rage that I figured out. Or I think I have figured out. If things like this can ever be figured out. This festered for two weeks between my November 2018 sessions with Dr. Plié. I think I was watching The Good Doctor, a TV show about an autistic man who grows up to be a surgical intern. Dear CBS, you are welcome for the plug. One scene triggered an insight into my situation. In the scene, the doctors pondered, "There were no similar symptoms for X number of years, or ever. Now we have this symptom out of the blue. Why is this happening?" And no one on my medical posse asked this question. Not one. Until I finally did. Regardless, my festering festered. Nothing would change, no matter how much I percolated about it. Plus, everything seemed to be working. Oh man, I shouldn't have written that.

THE QUADRUPLE WHAMMY OF 2018-2019
HAPPY BIRTHDAY MOM

2017 was comparatively uneventful health wise compared to the previous eight years. There were the usual couple of pacemaker glitches that lead to a couple of overnight hospital admissions, but no major events. Although Mom was starting to concern us. She was having spells and falling. I went to see her in January for her birthday. I had said goodbye to Mom, was back at the hotel, with a couple of hours before my return flight, I get a call from my cousin that the EMTs were with mom. Mom had fallen, hit her head and was being taken to emergency. She was in good spirits when I got to the hospital, but it would be a couple of hours before they could get her in for a CT scan. The doctor told me she was fine, just doing the CT as a precaution. I'm not sure how I knew this, but I sensed mom had had enough of the hospital at this point. She has a great sense of humour and is such a trooper. I rebooked my flight for a few hours later and after the CT gave the all clear, I headed to the airport.

My hands were still freezing, but overall, I seemed to be making progress. Although the progress is never linear or always forward. As I left the hospital for the airport, the wicked cold impaired my already freezing hands even more. So much so that even using the fob, I couldn't unlock the car. I had to get security to unlock the car. I am positive the guy thought I was pranking him or something. Even back in the milder Toronto winters, I've had times where I could barely unlock my bike lock. "Cold hands" is another one of those things that shouldn't be a major life impediment, but it can be. It's currently August 2022. I am sitting on the deck working. And my hands are experiencing yet another cold spell. My keyboarding speed is reduced dramatically. I wonder if we will ever get a hand-le on this?

ENTER INTERMITTENT FASTING

Then something happened that profoundly changed my life and the lives of many others I know. I mean beyond the impacts of my pacemakers and leads apparently being bought at the discount stores. It's suddenly Feb 2018 and I am waiting in an exam room for a regular check up with my cardiologist, Dr. Pedals (Just a reminder, he's a cyclist, so he pedals, not peddles). He walks into the room holding something behind his back and asks, "Has there been any time in your life you haven't been some level of obese?" Hi doc, nice to see you too! I respond, "Nope, always a chunky monkey or fat as far as I can remember. Just times I have been fairly fit from hockey and rugby but still obese". Then he pulls a book out from behind his back, throws it at me and says, "Buy this, read this, do this. After we coordinate with your other doctors, of course". The book was *The Obesity Code* by Dr. Jason Fung, a nephrologist based out of Toronto. Spoiler alert – and this is truly a life altering concept - the premise is that most obesity is not cured by the traditional CICO (calories in/calories out or exercise more/eat less models). And you don't fail on your diets because you suck or have no self-discipline or willpower. Most people are overweight because their gut biome/hormonal/metabolic systems are messed up. And hormones beat will power every minute of every hour of every day of every week and so on. And there is a way to get your gut biome/hormones rebalanced and get

THE SUMMER I DIED TWENTY TIMES

healthy again. And it's called Intermittent Fasting (IF). And the medical community has known about it for decades. The esteemed medical bible *New England Journal of Medicine* (NEJM) recently published an article on the benefits of Intermittent Fasting, particularly on longevity. It's in the December 26, 2019 edition. If Intermittent Fasting makes it into the NEJM, you know it's legit. There is going to be a lot about Intermittent Fasting woven into the story as we go forward. It is that important. You might even become an IF practitioner or coach after reading this.

It took a while for all the doctors to send letters to each other and to get together to work out if I could do this. Two months later, in early April 2018, I got the ok to give fasting a shot. I bought the book (again, *The Obesity Code*), read the book, and started to do the book. What is weird is that even though I've been overweight all my life and knew that diets don't work for most people long term, I didn't question the info in this book one bit. The science just made too much sense. Even knowing that fasting for tests or surgery or even Yom Kippur had been very difficult for me, I just went for it. To be honest, I expected it to be much harder than it was. Initially, like for maybe the first two weeks, the mental aspect was harder than the actual adhering to the fasting part. Overall, it was surprisingly easy. More often than not, it is the people I interacted with who were uncomfortable with my fasting and skipping meals than I was. Although not anymore. The evidence is pretty obvious IF works (wait until you read the riveting stories about my pants in the sequel) and they are used to me fasting. For the most part.

Initially, I remember more than a few meal invites where I just drank water and those around the table couldn't handle me not eating. Are you sure you don't want anything? Are you sure this is healthy? This can't be healthy. You must be hungry. How can you not be hungry? Thankfully, we are all past that now. Well, mostly. *The Obesity Code* made so much sense to me. Using its principles has healed my body in ways I couldn't imagine and still can't fully comprehend. I am so thrilled with the weight loss and healing from Intermittent Fasting (IF) that I now coach and give talks about it. I'll talk more about this later. Why not talk about it now, you ask? Ok, I will, a bit. But not much. Because I'm about to have another Fred "Kind of Day". In other words, do I have a story for you!

I haven't really fasted as an adult except for occasionally on Yom Kippur or for a blood test. And even in recent years, I wasn't even strict on Yom Kippur because of the medications I need having to be taken with food and liquid. Plus, given my medical history, the doctors and I had no clue how my body would react to Intermittent Fasting. I started off my IF journey conservatively, fasting (water only) for 12 hours, then having 12 hours to eat my three meals, then do the same thing the next day. And the next. And the next after that. In the IF world, they call this a 12:12 schedule. The format is "Fasting Window: Eating Window". My current daily schedule (2022) is generally a 20:4 or a 22:2 with two one longer fasts (38-42 hours) a week. And I feel great. In fact, better than I ever remember feeling. Later I will get into Non-Scale Victories. Suffice to say, that with my history, to be 59 years old and have zero body aches and the ability to cycle 90 minutes in the humidexes of 40 Celsius (104 Fahrenheit) blows my mind. Oh yeah, back to the Fred "Kind of Day".

THE BEGINNING OF THE END OF THE
BEGINNING 2.0

I was a week or so in on my IF journey and it was Saturday evening. April 21, 2018. I was walking home from Synagogue (Oh crap. Didn't we kind of start this adventure like this? Not again!) when I took a detour. I wanted to drop in on Statler and Waldorf, you know, the old curmudgeons from the Muppets. Actually, they are lovely old geezers and it had been far too long since I'd seen them. I knocked on their door, was pleasantly surprised that they were still ~~alive~~ awake, and we had a nice socially distanced visit on the porch. Actually, there was no social distancing needed. Maybe a foreshadowing of COVID-19 about 2 years early. We visited for an hour or so and I went on my merry way, about a 15-20-minute walk home. About 5 minutes into my journey, I had a minor brainquake. My knees buckled. I fell to one knee, but I didn't lose consciousness. I started sweating a bit and was a bit shaken. That seemed to be the extent of it. I had just been to the Pacemaker Clinic that week. Everything was as it should be. I probably should have learned by now not to be as confident in those analyses as I am. My next thought was, "Maybe this was some weird side effect of Intermittent Fasting?" I couldn't see how it could be related, but I was still new to the IF world and still didn't know all the intricacies yet. Maybe? Possibly? To be determined. Of course, now I know if I feel off, my first thought should always be...yep...pacemaker.

Monday was April 23rd (my birthday – wiring cash is my preferred gift if you are so inspired. Or buying copies of this book as gifts to others also works. Or both. Or sponsoring my podcast. You know the drill.) My mentioning this will make more sense a few paragraphs from now. A few days go by since the Saturday evening event, and I still feel a little off. Just to keep the timeline straight, it is now Thursday, April 26, 2018. I go to my regular appointment with Dr. Plié, which is to be followed with a physical at Dr. Coif's. It's a good hour travel between their offices. Dr. Plié and I go through all our regular reporting, after which I tell her what happened. As soon as I finish telling her everything, Boom! Another minor brainquake. Thankfully, I was sitting in a good position and didn't fall over. "It just happened again". Dr. Plie responded "Yes, I could tell something just happened. We should wrap up and you should get to Dr. Coif right away". Why didn't Dr. Plié check me out herself you ask? Even though she is a fully trained MD, psychiatrists generally aren't stocked with the traditional doctor accoutrements like stethoscopes, thermometers, blood pressure cuffs, etc. There was nothing she could check me with. I grabbed a ride share. Hey ride share company: I'd give you a plug if you want to work out some sort of product placement or promotional deal. Free luxury ride share for life is a good starting place. Ride shares are amazing. It's like going on a mini-trip to another country. On the ride, I learned all about my ride share driver's adventures in Culinary School, including how he worked on cruise ships developing his own style of modern fusion something something. I don't really understand what fusion cooking is. Between how I was feeling and his accent, I couldn't figure out what the something something was. I suspect it was cuisine from the area he grew up in. Anyhow, he has his dream to open his own restaurant. I hope it works out for him. Who knows? It's been a couple of years. Maybe it already has!

Traffic was on our side and with my cutting Dr. Plie's appointment short, I arrived well before my scheduled appointment with Dr. Coif. The receptionist noted I did not look good (yep, the staff sees me far too often), then messaged the doctor. He came out to the waiting room, looked at me and said, "Go to the hospital". I call the ride share again. I know, I know. You are thinking if I looked so bad, why didn't he call an ambulance for me? Unfortunately, our ambulance system works in zones. They take you to the nearest hospital and he wanted me at the hospital with my entire history and the doctors who had worked on me. I am certain that if he thought I was past a certain level of danger, he would have called an ambulance to get me to the hospital about 5 blocks away.

In the ride share (again ride share companies, same offer as above), I realized this might turn into an overnight visit, so I decided to stop at home to grab my go bag. I quickly learned that unlike a traditional taxi that you can reroute at anytime, ride share people don't like to reroute because they don't know how to figure out the change in charges. Thankfully, this has since changed so you can book multi-stage rides. Although if you don't prearrange it on the app, you get dinged with an additional booking fee. A $20 cash settlement fee later, I am at home grabbing my stuff. As we are leaving, I see a neighbour leaving another neighbour's house. Although we only lived about seven houses apart around the corner, with her hubby and her living there for over 30 years, we'd only formally met maybe a week ago. We'd seen each other many times but had never talked or been introduced. "A ride share?" she teased me. "I think this is the first time I've seen you going somewhere without your bike or walking". I said, "Believe me, I wish I was on my bike right now". I didn't see her again until the late fall of 2020. I think to this day, she doesn't know what happened.

DO YOU SWEAR TO TELL THE TRUTH, THE WHOLE TRUTH AND NOTHING BUT THE TRUTH?

It is around 5 PM at this point. I get to the all too familiar emergency unit and try to explain what is going on. I must have looked like total crap by this point as they triaged me (took down all my history etc.) while doing the ECG and blood draws. They keep saying I am obviously having a heart attack because I am sweating a lot. I respond I am sweating a lot because I am wearing two jackets – part of my go bag collection. It is often pretty chilly in the hospital, so I bring extra clothes. They ignore my reasoning and put me straight into a room with a continuous heart monitor. Eventually, Doctor Team number one comes in (a doctor and a resident or newbie) and I relay how I have had problems with my pacemakers, I've just started IF, the recent brainquakes, etc. They don't seem to believe my story. I say well, it's all in my file. Call Dr. Kugel, Dr. Pedals, or the Pacemaker Clinic. "Uh, no". they respond. "We're not going to bother them with this". It is confirmed. They don't believe me and are not taking me seriously at all. Wash, rinse, repeat. A couple of hours later, Doctor Team number two comes in. They ask all the same questions. It's like a court scene in a Law or Police procedural drama. A witness is on the stand testifying and the opposing attorney or prosecutor is intent on catching them in a lie, instead of getting to the truth. The blood vampires come by again to drain a few quarts. Around 10 PM, a nurse comes in. She brings me my medications; tells me they are keeping me overnight and are actually going to admit me to the cardiac ward. That is, as soon as a bed is available. Again, I must give props to the nurses and all the frontline staff. They do an amazing job. I say to her "Well, they must have some suspicions about something then". She responds "Not that anyone has relayed to us. Your logic seems right. If they are keeping you, they definitely think something is going on because the cardiac ward is full. It will be a while until we can transfer you". Around midnight, the blood vampires come again. Thankfully, the hospital made a dramatic upgrade to the Wi-Fi system, and I can stream movies on my laptop. I sleep a little bit, then a third doctor comes in. An Internal Medicine doctor I believe. After she asks me the first couple of cross-examination questions, I get annoyed. Probably more tired than annoyed. Naw, I'll stick with annoyed. I ask her why they take these notes, bring the file to the room with them, then no one reads the notes. And we keep going through this. Just read the damn notes. It's a simple concept. Apparently, no one has even mentioned this basic premise to the good Doctor. She is not happy. Shocker, she reads the notes in the chart "Your pacemaker has failed previously and been replaced? Not a normal occurrence". "Yes", I reply. "There have been many complications". She doesn't respond. Then. She. Just. Turns. Around. And. Leaves. I never saw her again.

I'm guessing it is about 3 AM when one of the orderlies wakes me. "Time to go, Sir. We have a bed for you. Are you able to walk yourself?" I say yes, the Nurse (in slightly more colourful language) says not a chance. I repack my go bag and off we go on a gurney ride. Quick tangent. I'm not sure what it is about gurney rides or having people watch as you get placed in an ambulance, but I find it quite embarrassing. I wonder if others do too. Something else to explore with Dr. Plié. We finally get to the Cardiac Ward and to my room. Looking through the door, I see it is a dorm room. Six beds stuffed into a room for four. It is obviously over-crowded. This is the first time I've not been in a one or two-person room. "How will I be able to sleep with all this going on?" I wonder. The guy beside me and another guy are medalists in Olympic snoring. Another guy is a perpetual screamer. And no personal space. Now I know I have my flaws as a room mate, but as Dr. Pedals says, "A hospital is a horrible place for sick people". I ask the nurse where my call bell is. Oh, we don't have one for your bed. I'll get you something. Something?

What she brings back is this – an old school hotel-desk type service bell. I guess I can take reservations, book people into their rooms and call for bellhops while I recover. My understanding is doing this bell thing, never mind the entire room overcrowding, is not exactly up to code. So randomly weird. Anyhow, I decide to make the best of things. Much to my amazement, I unpacked, got settled, and slept for a couple of hours. Guess who woke me up? Well, it wasn't the blood vampire coming for the 6 AM blood drain. It was my immediate neighbour's wife, who woke her hubby as soon as she arrived. You know it is early when you beat the blood vampires. Even though they deprived me of a few more minutes of sleep, I thought it was quite touching that this woman made such an effort to be the first thing her husband saw in the morning. I am guessing they are in their late 60s, maybe a touch older. She was there from roughly 6 AM to 7 PM every day. Now, English was not their first language, so sometimes I couldn't quite follow all our chats. I'm just going to call them Mr. and Mrs. Med, as they came from somewhere in the Mediterranean. Mrs. Med told me, or at least this is what I understood, that she married Mr. Med, sight unseen, in an arranged marriage. He had already moved to Canada when she was sent here to be his bride. I also thought she said Mr. Med was just a hard-working masonry guy. Mr. Med was 100% bedridden. Me, well, beyond walking the hallways in our area or the odd visit to the lounge, I was also pretty much confined to bed. One way I tried to alleviate my boredom was by taking advantage of the diversity of the nursing staff. They are from all over the world, so I began asking them if their names had any meanings. You know, as opposed to my name, which, to the best of my knowledge, has no specific meaning. Many played along. And some names were fascinating: Moon Princess, Celestial Voyageur, Warrior of Peace. I'd ask them silly questions, like: What are the duties of a Moon Princess? Do Celestial Voyageurs get Air Miles? That would be sweet! A Warrior of Peace fights for the little guy. I wish I could remember more of them.

Later that afternoon, one of the Med's sons came for a visit. Son and dad started talking about investment properties, leveraging, market demand, whether they wanted property X anymore. I was fascinated by this. Obviously, he wasn't just a simple labourer. I wondered why they weren't talking in their native language. Papa Med later said the kids were born in Canada, so they made their kids learn English first. The kids barely speak their parent's language at all. Momma Med sat dutifully by them. I have no idea if she understood any of this financial talk.

Given it's Saturday and the Jewish Sabbath, I didn't expect any calls or visitors. I hadn't told many people I was back in the hospital. It was going to be a pretty chill day. In my experience, not a lot of testing/diagnosing goes on in the hospital on the weekends. More the emergency stuff seems to be the priority. The Pacemaker Clinic is closed on the weekends, so I knew I wasn't having anything done. So, it surprised me when they came and took Papa Med off for some tests. Mama Med either didn't understand what the tests were or couldn't communicate it to me. I tried to get some sleep but the gentleman screamer in the room was still going strong. Dementia/Alzheimer's or whatever was afflicting him is a horrible thing. From what he kept screaming, he had been in a POW camp. Tragic that he went through this torture once. Now he is going through it again and again on a continuous loop. I hope he found peace. I fell asleep, so of course, so you know what that means – a visit from the blood vampires and/or a nurse to take your vitals. And conveniently, I had another episode of some sort while the nurse was there. And more conveniently, I was still in bed and didn't fall or crack my head again. I hate these things happening to me but am grateful when they happen with credible witnesses.

THE INCEL INCIDENT

You be wondering why I am sharing so much about my room mates, the Meds. There are two reasons. One, it's a thread that will show up again in the future (Jan 2020). Two, remember I mentioned my birthday date a few paragraphs ago? (Still waiting on those cash transfers. Just saying). It turns out April 23, 2018, is also the date of the terrible incident in a Toronto neighbourhood when an Incel man killed a number of people and injured many others. Mostly women, with a rented Van. Just awful. You can search Incels if you aren't familiar with the term. And why do I mention this tragic, obscure event? A couple of reasons. I rode my bike through the same area a few hours after the event, saw all the police and emergency services up and down the street. Naively, I thought they were doing an emergency response training drill. It's not unusual to see them drilling in one of the Toronto subway stations or in a mall. And until writing this down, I didn't even process that I had been at that horrific spot. Second, the Meds live in that area. Momma Med had been out that day and barely avoided being run down. So with that and Papa Med having who knows what going on, it's already been a pretty awful week for Mama Med. Now adding on waiting for the test results until some time next week.

Sunday comes and word gets out that I am in the hospital again. Visitors are trickling in. I have a couple more mini episodes, so it's also the first time anyone in my inner circle sees what's happening to me. Thankfully, these are nothing like my previous full on brainquake spasming episodes. And also thankfully, they brought me some books, quality food and Mrs. Phelps (like the Olympic swimmer), who brought me some toiletries when she was already time crunched. I am not sure what happened to the toiletry kit in my go bag, but somehow it went somewhere. Also appreciative to my buddy Data (like the character in Star Trek) who brought me a specific type of candy I was craving (Do I even need to say it? Product placement opportunities are available!)

SCREW THE FOOD GUIDES, HOSPITAL FOOD AND DIABETES

To the extent that I could, I was still trying to fast while in the hospital. Hospital policy disagrees with this. Even when they come to take your meal requests for the day, and I tell them I have food or don't want anything, they still bring you a tray. So wasteful. And don't get me started on the quality of food or basing the nutrition on the Food Guides, which more and more people are realizing are total agenda driven BS. And the people in the hospitals are complicit in this. And dieticians and doctors. Given that I am (or was) type 2 diabetic, foods low in sugars are the best thing for me. I say was because via Intermittent Fasting, my blood sugars are now consistently in the normal range. But try getting the diabetic label off your medical chart. UGH! You beat cancer and you are a survivor, cancer free. You get your blood sugar numbers down to normal, you are no longer diabetic. Except to doctors and medical charts. You are always diabetic. I don't get it.

Anyhow, the dieticians, at least the ones I have dealt with, insist that as a type 2 diabetic, you need 45 grams of carbs per meal. If you don't know, carbs are, for the most part a fancy word for refined sugar. Which blows right through you and raises your blood sugar. Versus complex carbs which are natural or much less refined and don't blow right through you. They give you "low" sugar foods like those breakfast cereals, which the companies boldly claim are low sugar. Only 3 grams, honest! Would we lie or deceive you? Of course not! We are a huge multinational food company. We are your moral compass. Breakfast is the most important meal of the day (said no scientific body ever). What the food company doesn't say is that the cereal I was being served is actually 23 grams of carbs (aka sugar). But the labelling guidelines allow them to separate the direct sugar from the refined carbs to fool readers. Be aware. Food labels can be deceptive. If I decide to go on another rant, I'll add in the evils of processed vegetable oils. Or talk about how supplements are for the most part a scam. Read this article in the LA Times about how a certain Senator facilitated allowing supplement companies to sell snake oil with no oversight. https://www.latimes.com/business/hiltzik/la-fi-hiltzik-hatch-20180105-story.html. And people wonder why we have a cardiac, obesity, diabetes and metabolic crises going on right now.

ENTER INDIANA JONES AND THE ARTIFACTS

I'm possibly going to go all Neil deGrasse Tyson on you. Ok, maybe Bill Nye. Or Sheldon Cooper. Fine, more Leonard Hoeffsteder than Sheldon. I'm guessing most of you have seen a regular ECG reading, either your own or on some fake heart monitor on a medical show. Mine generally don't show much beyond that I seem to be alive because the pacemaker produces a regular controlled signal. Or at least that is what it normally does when it isn't failing. Unless the reading is taken at the exact moment, the pacemaker fails (like when my Holter monitor caught it in 2009), you don't see anything that gives you any new insights.

NORMAL ECG 1

Except there was something unusual on my readings. Something that would make Indiana Jones excited. No, not like the Ark of the Covenant. But there were artifacts. Lots and lots of artifacts. Artifacts are crazy readings that sometimes show up, often overlaying the regular ECG. They can present themselves in a number of ways. For me, they showed up like a 4-year-old trying to colour between the lines. And it was continuous. Or so they thought. This should have been a huge red flag. I mean, I can see the difference. Can you see the difference? Unfortunately, no one asked – why after 8 years of never seeing one artifact, was I now producing copious amounts of them? I mean, isn't that a question that would occur to you? Of course it would. But not to the 5-10 medical professionals on my case.

My attending nurse (I had a hard time choosing what to call her. It was between Nurse Beaver – she could gnaw down a tree, or Nurse Helium – what an annoying voice). I just went with the combo celebrity-type name Nurse Belium (think Bennifer/Brangelina). Belium told me she had extensive special training in reading artifacts. She said she showed them to the Dr. in charge. I will call him Dr. Infomercial because he had that smile and voice style that screamed late night infomercial. And if you order now, we will not only give you not one misdiagnosis, not two misdiagnoses, but three misdiagnoses! And if you call in the next 10 minutes, we will throw in the world's smallest juicer.

Nurse Belium and Dr. Infomercial concluded with not much investigation that the artifacts were just reading me moving around, and it was no big deal. But I knew this couldn't be true because I was having varying degrees of syncopes. Just prior to the syncopes, I could feel my heart gurgle. My best description is if you have ever had a car stall on a wintry day and you try to crank it. It spurts and sputters and struggles to start. I decided every time I felt one of these incidents, I would record it and what I was doing. Of course, I was in the hospital and was not allowed off the ward. The large majority of my time was sitting or lying-in bed, you know, not moving around.

A heart can easily beat 100,000 times a day. Based on what I know now, my heart was stopping to some degree 150 – 200 times a day. Roughly 8 times per hour. Some of these stops were quite significant, others were too subtle to notice. Yesterday (Aug 12, 2018, about 3.5 months post-surgery), I went for a walk in Edward's Gardens with Rabbi Chili Burger and her family. If you ever have time to visit the Gardens, take it. Incredibly beautiful tranquil place. The Burgers and I were climbing a moderately inclined stone stairway of maybe 15 steps. When we got to the top, I had no breath. I knew immediately I had a significant heart stoppage. I dropped to my knees in case a full syncope happened. Thankfully, it didn't. I was no worse for wear, except for some dirty knees. These incidents really mess with your mind. There is perpetual anxiety that the pacemaker can fail, anytime, anywhere.

I took the gurgle list to Nurse Belium and told her what I did. She responded so what; the artifacts are all background noise. I insisted. Strongly. Look at each recorded time and check what my heart is doing. We went over and went through the ECG strips. It was obvious there were significant artifacts at every time I listed. Nurse Belium got confused because I obviously couldn't be moving around so much to cause all these artifacts. Then I suggested (probably more than a little smugly) that they need to go through my strips again because something was obviously causing my heart to misfire and stop. I mean, I was admitted to the cardiac ward because they suspected something was going wrong. If you get a lead (no pacemaker pun intended), check it out.

Even though she was very annoyed/upset with me for not playing the good follow-the-medical-people-blindly patient, she called Dr. Infomercial. The body language was fascinating. Much like when a puppy knows it's getting scolded. Or when a little kid is busted but keeps telling Mommy and Daddy they didn't eat any cake – even though their face is covered in chocolate. Anyhow, Doc Infomercial finally showed up to take a look, and was not pleased. He comes to my room and admits something is wrong with the pacemaker and we will need to explore further. And yet, I still don't have a medical degree. Mind blowing.

Not to state the obvious, but why didn't it occur to anyone that seeing as I had zero artifacts (that anyone shared with me) in the previous nine years, suddenly having them show up in large amounts meant something had changed. Seems pretty obvious to me.

THE TEAM FINALLY PUTS THEIR FINGER ON IT

Thankfully, I had a ton of visitors for this hospital stay. For the most part, Dr. Kugel was frustrated. Something was going on, but we just couldn't put our fingers on it. Until we did. Literally. Kugel asked his fellow pacemaker specialist, Dr. Ravioli, for his opinion. They brought the pacemaker clinic gadgets into my room. Let's see if we can recreate what causes these artifacts. We want you to twist and turn and try to mimic any movement you might make in bed. Holy crap. Right on cue, certain movements showed the artifacts. For the next steps, Dr. Ravioli literally put his fingers on it. He started manipulating the pacemaker with his hands, pushing it around at different angles and watching the artifacts show up. Then it happened. He hit the perfect spot and brainquake; I was gone again. But only briefly. As soon as they saw what was happening, Ravioli stopped manipulating the pacemaker. That was far less unpleasant than normal. Here we go again folks. Another pacemaker lead failed. What to do next? Good question. This would take some figuring out, for sure.

Kugel and Ravioli consulted with other pacemaker doctors. Along with consulting with Dr. Pedals and other internal staff, the plan was hatched. Leave the original pacemaker alone at first. It sat on the left side of my chest. Insert a new pacemaker and two new leads on the right side of my chest, get it up and running, then turn off the malfunctioning left side pacemaker off so it never bothers me again. It seemed like the simplest fix. Easy peasy. At some point if we need to, all the old wiring could be removed via a separate procedure called a lead extraction surgery. The lead extraction is a pretty low risk procedure but not entirely risk free. We'll deal with that when we need to. For now, we were starting from scratch. What could go wrong? I mean, we aren't even going near the collapsed vein, defective pacemaker, and defective leads. Right?

It took a few days to arrange a surgery spot. Every day, a new gaggle of med students would come by to see how moving my pacemaker could make me syncope. Nothing like an extra six or eight people into my already overcrowded room to further inconvenience me and my roomies. Mr. Med had gotten a grim diagnosis. Mrs. Med said her brother had died from the same thing. Obviously, she was pretty shaken. I reminded her that was maybe 40 years ago, and treatments here today are so much better than in small Mediterranean towns back then. I don't think that helped. Emma the pacemaker Queen comes by to tell me they arranged a surgery slot, all the parts have been ordered and we are good to go. I joked "I hope you didn't order from one of those 99 cent stores again". Then I asked if she could get Dr. Kugel to come by or let me know when he was in clinic as I had a request for him. A few hours later, Kugel comes by. You have some questions? "Actually, more a couple of requests. One primary request". Kugel responds "Ok, this is interesting. Ask away". I respond, "I want to be put under a general anesthetic for the procedure. No locals. I want to be fully out". Kugel scrunched up his face. "We'd prefer not to just for safety and recovery reasons. Why do you want to do this?" "Well, I am sure you remember what happened my first surgery. Possibly you don't know this, but the follow up surgery was also a total shit show. If by cosmic freak, this goes bad again, I don't want to be aware of it. I just don't need anything else adding PTSD to my life. I've had enough". "I understand. I didn't know about the problems with the second surgery. Totally reasonable request on your part. Let me talk to Pedals and see if we can arrange an anesthetist at this short notice. As soon as I know, you will know". And the wheels were set in motion.

UP IN SMOKE

The next couple of days were kind of chill. The screaming man went to another ward, so everyone slept better. Another patient replaced him. A relatively young man. He claimed he didn't speak English, but I suspected he did. Don't ask me why I suspected this. I just did. Every time anyone needed to talk to him, they had to call for a translator, then wait for the translator, then talk to the patient. Ooops. Scratch that. The guy was on his cellphone constantly. The drill was actually, call the translator, wait for the translator, wait for the guy to acknowledge them, wait until he finished his call, then talk to him. Super time consuming. Often while waiting for the translator, the guy would just walk away. He'd disconnect his heart monitor and snuck out to have a smoke. If I could figure this out, not sure why no one else could. The doctor/translator told him his heart arteries were almost totally clogged, he had to stop smoking immediately and he for sure couldn't smoke for 24 hours before his surgery. The doctor sternly told him if he didn't have the surgery, he would be dead by year's end. They left, off comes the monitor, and he's off for another great smoke escape. I wish I knew what happened to him, but when I returned from my procedure, he was gone. Oh yes, my procedure. What? You forgot I was having another procedure? But now that you remember, you think this will take place incident free? Not a chance. I told the Meds my surgery was the next day.

I wasn't sure if they were bringing me back to this hospital or I would recover at the other hospital. I said a prayer for them, not knowing if I would ever see them again.

The Transport Ambulance guys show up and off we go. The doctors told me to fast from about 10 PM on. I could have liquids only. What they were supposed to say was clear liquids. I have been through the drill and should have known this. The next day, Dr. Kugel was less than pleased to see me drinking one of those artificially sweetened beverages where you squeeze a few drops into your water. But we hugged it out, and all was good. I was again fascinated by the diversity of the staff, especially the meanings of their names and origin stories. My attending nurse was Bulgarian (I'll call her B1). I think I know two other Bulgarians – a pharmacist and a woman (I'll call her B2) I met through, well, I don't actually remember how we met. But I will message her and get back to you. I am sure it is a fascinating story. I think B2 told me a tale of how her grandfather or great-grandfather was Jewish and somehow became a high-ranking officer of an Eastern European church. Or maybe the head of the church. Anyhow, B1 said she didn't know many Bulgarians, my friend didn't either, so I thought, hey, let's connect them. I dialled up B2, told her what was going on, then passed the phone to B1. They had a lovely chat while I was getting prepped for surgery. In the middle, the anesthetist (Dr. Sleep) came by. Dr. Sleep told me what was going to happen: some anti-asthma medicine, some antihistamine, some anti-anxiety stuff, and all should be good. Then it was time to get manscaped. I'm telling you, those electric shavers they have are top of the line. I should have grabbed one for home use, as I suspect they are priced at the very top of the market.

PACEMAKER REPLACEMENT ATTEMPT 3 –
YET ANOTHER CLUSTERFUCK

It was finally time. I got my meds. Another gurney ride begins. Today's gurney driver's name translated to Mighty, as in Mighty Warrior. We arrived at the lab, and I remembered how icey cold these things were. By the time we get set up, it's roughly 12:30 PM. Dr. Sleep does her magic. The show begins. Next thing I know, I'm on my way back to recovery. Even being barely conscious, I recognize I am not a happy camper. I am trying to clear my head. The drugs won't let me. And the more I try, the more irritated I get. Initially, I thought I was one of those people who have trouble clearing out the general anesthetic. Lots of people are like this and are often quite crabby. Again, I said initially. Then I notice it's like 5:00 PM. 5 PM? What happened to my 30-minute procedure? Even in my distressed state, I clue in. Aw shit, something went wrong in the surgery. Again! I was having so much trouble clearing out the anesthetic because they had to use so much on me for way longer than expected. My apologies to the nurses – I suspect I was a total dick trying to get the drugs out of my system. It was around 8 PM when I finally seemed to clear out. I had a new nursing crew with Anastasia (you'll meet her again later) being my primary nurse. As my surgery had run long, combined with it taking me so long to wake up, I was now 20 hours fasted. And hungry. Except they had no food for me as I was supposed to have been returned to Hospital "A" hours ago. I was supposed to eat at Hospital A but any dinner there was long gone. Anastasia had no clue what happened in the surgery, why it took so long and why I was put out so deeply. She put in a call to the transport service, who weren't answering the phones. Weird. I alternated between walking up and down the ward (maybe 100 feet round trip) and trying to lie down and chill. Maybe around 9:30, there was a massive flash of lightning, an enormous clap of thunder, and the lights flickered hard. Oh crap, we were having a super cell storm. These storms hit different parts of the city at different times. And they hit hard. There weren't a lot of ground level windows on the ward, but through the upper windows we could see the tops of trees bending sideways. Certainly, we could see the relentless lightning and hear the thunder, wind and driving rain. Now we understood why the transport ambulances weren't picking up. It was probably bedlam trying to drive anywhere in the city.

These types of storms blow through quickly. The ward was pretty empty and the odds of anyone one else joining us were pretty low. Finally, Anastasia connected with the transport crew – they'd be another couple of hours. Plus, they needed a three-person crew, as I was like five pounds over the weight limit for a two-man crew. I was confused. I was brought in by a two-man crew with no problems. Had the new pacemaker put me over the top? Who knows? It certainly didn't feel that heavy. And I know it wasn't from me overeating because there was no food to overeat. Companies and their weird rules. They finally arrived around 2:30 in the morning and off we went. Oh, and the 3rd guy on the crew? Did absolutely nothing. Good thing we waited. We did chat about him wanting a new bike. I advised him to go for a hybrid with the new disc brakes. They finally got me back to my ward. I was too tired to eat. The nurse literally tucked me in. I wish I had a do not disturb sign to hang on my door. Actually, I wish I had a door to my room period. Before I knew it, it was 6

AM and time to draw blood and check my vitals. I was so tired. Just let me rest and come back in 8 hours. No? Didn't think so. Mrs. Med came in. Sweetheart that she is, wanted to make sure I was ok. I fell asleep talking to her. I woke around nine AM to my delicious breakfast, which was soon followed by Drs. Pedals and Kugel. "Good morning, sunshine. Well, we have some good news and some less than good news".

BECOMING THE
EIGHTH WONDER OF THE WORLD

"So here is the good news. You are now the proud owner of two simultaneously functioning pacemakers". Wait, what? Two what? "The bad news is we weren't able to install both leads for the new pacemaker. But we did get the more important one in. After a couple of hours of struggle and consulting, we've set you up so that when the malfunctioning pacemaker glitches, the new one will sense it and kick in". Pedals chimed in, "At some point, we'll have to do a more permanent solution as the old battery only has so many years left on it (I think it had 4 years projected lifespan at this point). But for now, this keeps you up and running. Be thankful you had someone as creative as Dr. Kugel working on you". No one explained why they couldn't get the new pacemaker fully installed. I muttered something like "Well, that explains the anesthetic overdose". "Yeah, sorry about that. But in the end, it was still good that we went that route". Then a third voice chimed in, "We need to go to Rounds and explain your situation. Very few people in the world are being kept alive by concurrent pacemakers". Rounds - versus the doctors making rounds to visit patients - are special staff meetings where unusual situations or cases are presented. My understanding is I have been the feature presentation in Rounds a few times. In the subsequent adventures trying to find a workable solution to my situation, one doctor told me I am one of only eight people in the world who have two pacemakers running concurrently. That makes me the new eighth wonder of the world. Every doctor I've met since initially doesn't believe that I am running on two pacemakers, then reluctantly believes I have two, but that only one can be functioning. Then I get the "Lots of patients have one live pacemaker and even a couple of dead pacemakers that were just not taken out" responses. Ultimately, they read my chart and finally come around to believing me. What possible reason could I have for making this up? Maybe I will make it past Rounds and will get a write up in the New England Journal of Medicine. Assuming this works, that is. Hey! New England Journal of Medicine. Call me.

MEET THE CONTRARIANS

I spent the next couple of days chilling. Cassie and Dr. Beatles came into town and got me home, helped clean my apartment. It really was quite a disaster – cleaning, tidying, and organizing hasn't been a priority. And honestly, it's never been something I excelled at. I have no evidence of this, but I believe this lifetime of head trauma has pretty much also knocked any cleaning genes I may have inherited completely out of my DNA. Check that. We know many who suffer from severe depression often have trouble keeping their spaces clean. My cleaning challenge is definitely something I always have to stay mindful of. They also shlepped me to a couple of doctor appointments. Thankfully, they no longer put your arm in a tight sling to protect the stitches and leads. Remember, this new pacemaker was inserted in my upper right chest, so historically, I would have had my right arm in the sling. As I've mentioned, my left side of my body doesn't work really well, so having my left arm/hand as my only functioning appendages is not much help. It allowed me to help with the apartment clean up to some degree. Maybe help is an exaggeration.

While that was going on, I had friends (The Contrarians) insist that I stay with them while my apartment was getting straightened out. Well, Mrs. Contrarian insisted. She loves hosting dinners and guests. Mr. Contrarian didn't buy in so much, but generally goes along for the ride with Mrs. C's decisions. I enjoy their company.

Together, they make a pretty balanced couple. If Mrs. C said I was staying, I was staying. I think I stayed for nine days. I should note that Mr. Contrarian is only contrarian for his own amusement. If you are pro-religion, he takes an anti-religion stance. If you are conservative, he'll go liberal. If you think taxes should go up, he'll be for tax-relief. I've watched him pull off this chameleon routine on countless unsuspecting ~~victims~~ guests. Including taking on guests from both sides of the aisle at the same time. It was super convenient staying there. A three-minute walk to synagogue. Literally across the street from the Borsalinos. It also guaranteed a regular flow of visitors. Which was both helpful and exhausting. I tried to make the best of my recuperating time by rereading *The Obesity Code* (or TOC, as the cool kids call it) and doing a first read *of The Big Fat Surprise: Why Butter, Meat and Cheese Belong in a Healthy Diet* by Nina Teicholz. I went through TOC again but never made it to Nina's book. Sorry Nina. Hopefully, I will get to it. It's for sure on my wait list at the library. I'm very grateful to the Contrarians and so many others who helped and continue to help me out.

DR. STEREOTYPE AND THE EXTENSION CORD SOLUTION

Dr. Kugel didn't waste any time looking into what options were available to tidy up my situation. It took maybe 10 days to get into another cardiac specialist at one of the downtown hospitals. You try to go into these meetings optimistically and with an open mind. At least I do. I'm waiting in, where else, the waiting room, doing some people watching. Once again, I am totally fascinated by the guy sitting across from me. I wonder if he has any clue of the impact he has on people. I so wanted to take a selfie with him. Him being another guy with a pornstache. It was so mesmerising that I didn't hear the receptionist call me for my appointment. Finally, I heard her and went into the exam room where the pacemaker tech introduced himself. And almost instantly, a partner joined him. I believe one was training or over seeing the other. I sat in the exam room for maybe 30 minutes. You know what I did? Same thing that always happens. I went over every question, note, and incident in my file with the technicians, who were pre-screening me. UGH. You have my files. You have letters from Dr. Pedals and Kugel. Read them for crying out loud. I wanted Cassie to listen in on the appointment with the new doctor. I called her and left her on speaker, waiting for the doctor to arrive. This time, there was no click click click of stilettos coming down the hall. Nor the sounds of angels singing when the door opened. Definitely not a VS model like the Ventricle Whisperer. Nor as nice. Have you ever seen a character in a TV show or movie that from their first appearance, you just know they are 100% unlikeable or next level arrogant? Well, meet Dr. Stereotype. He just sits down and starts talking to the pacemaker techs, doesn't even acknowledge me. The techs brief him, then he dismisses them. Finally, he gets around to me. "I'm Dr. Stereotype. Seems they (Kugel et al.) have you in a situation. Let's see what we can do". Thanks. Mind if my sister listens in? This is the moment he totally owns the arrogance and condescension. "Sure, but I doubt she'll understand anything. This is pretty high-level stuff". I reply "Well, she's been a high-end nurse longer than you've been a doctor. Plus, she testifies as a legal expert in malpractice cases. I think she can follow what's going on". "Oh, I didn't mean to infer that..." Uh, yeah, you certainly meant to infer something less than nice. Never mind doc, let's just move on. To my absolute surprise, he actually starts reading the file, then asks rhetorically, "Why didn't they just reset the (original) pacemaker settings to compensate for the issue? That would fix it". I asked, "What do you think they should have reset it to?" "Would you even know what I'm talking about?" "Try me and find out". Today I wouldn't have a chance at remembering any of the settings. But then, I still membered these conversations with Dr. Kugel and Ravioli. We spent a couple of hours together looking at alternatives. Pacemakers have many software packages to address a variety of conditions, so the doctors can choose which program to run to best help the patient. He was being a douche, so I decided he needed to know this wasn't appropriate. He names off an alternative setting. They tried that one, and it didn't help. We play this game a couple more times. He can't believe that I know this stuff – although in the current timeframe (June 2021), all that knowledge has disappeared. Finally, he proclaims, "I've got it. Use setting whatever". I said you can't. He asks why not? I said it's not part of this unit's software bundle. Of course, it is.

"No, it was discontinued about 3 years ago. In fact, we had a conference call with the pacemaker company and talked about just downloading the software. The pacemaker engineers said it was a no go". "I don't believe that. I'm going to go talk to my tech team". And Dr. Stereotype leaves for maybe 15 minutes. A visibly upset Dr. Stereotype comes back into the room (and to this day, I don't fully understand how this would help). "Here's what we can do. We can run a secondary lead from one pacemaker to the other to bypass the failure. But we really have to open you up to do this". Ok, I will talk to Kugel and Pedals and see what they think. "Well, don't take too long. It takes a while to get on the list here".

It takes a few weeks for things to get processed between Dr. Stereotype, Kugel, and Pedals. I have a follow up with Pedals at the end of June 2018. Pre-appointment, he sends me for a chest x-ray. I'm sitting in the exam room. I'm nervous – last time he threw a book at me! Peddles comes in, holding the x-ray. "You have to see this". He slaps it up on the light screen and laughs, "My friend, if you had any more wiring in you, we could just add a few light bulbs and you will never need a menorah for Channukah". I guess I never really thought about how much wire was running in and around my heart. I am guessing maybe eight feet worth. Each pacemaker lead is roughly 60 centimetres or two feet long. At that point, I had four leads in me. Side note: I had to go for more x-rays last week (Mid Aug 2020). The tech looks at the first image and says "Whoa! What is going on here? In 25 years, I've never seen so much wiring!" I've had some extra added since that meeting with Pedals – it's not quite a junkyard, but I am probably up to 12 feet now. Back to the matter at hand. Pedals says in his opinion, what Stereotype suggested is a no go. "Essentially, he wants to fix a glitchy pacemaker wire by making it into an extension cord. I don't know about your experiences with extension cords, but in my experience, they tend to disconnect and glitch themselves. So yes, people use this technique. It's not a risk we want to subject you to". Do the two of you have a suggestion?

"Yes, we mentioned this to you right after the operation, but who knows what you remember from then. You were still pretty out of it. This is longer term. When the older pacemaker gets near the end of its battery life, we'll potentially send you for a lead extraction procedure. It's not without risks, but it's less risky than the extension cord. Basically, they use a laser to release all the pacemaker leads from your heart. We remove them all and start everything from scratch. Or if you have a few hundred thousand dollars lying around, you can go to a place like the Cleveland Clinic and get it done there within weeks".

APOLOGIES TO THE CITY OF PAIN

"Well, if I go to Cleveland, I can hit up the Rock & Roll Hall of fame, maybe the Football Hall of Fame in Canton, then do the surgery. Or maybe catch an NFL game. Oh wait, they only have the Browns – not sure they qualify as an NFL team anymore. But whoever they play likely qualifies. (That was for you, KKC). I just have to work on getting that few hundred thousand to finance the deal. I guess I'll have to wait." Pedals continued, "Look, we know this isn't a perfect solution. There may still be some glitches, some syncopes in the meantime. So just be aware and if anything feels off, get to the hospital, ok?" Yessir! Off I went to resume (I hoped) getting back to my recovery and my life back on track.

THE VALLEY OF THE SHADOW OF DEATH

We move forward to September 2018. I have a double header today. Seeing Dr. Pedals and then off to the pacemaker clinic. I've done this ride before. It's probably a 7/10 on the exertion level, with a couple of significant hills (well, significant for me). The first one is what I call the Valley of Death. A lot of experienced riders on their $5000 bikes find it a challenge as well. But lately, I've been able to make it to the other side of the valley without stopping. But not this time. I didn't even make it halfway. I was huffing and puffing. I finally got to the top of the hill, sat for a bit, and caught my breath. I said to myself, "Sometimes, even the best athletes just don't have it that day. I'll keep going and see how far I can go. If I can't keep going, I'll just call a ride share or hop the subway". I wasn't really worried as I hadn't had a brainquake or anything. Off I went, plodding along at maybe half speed. At some point, I did a calculation, realizing that I wasn't going to be any sort of on time at this pace. The only solution was to head to the subway line, lock up my bike, hop on the subway and then walk up the hill to the medical building. I've done the hill many times, both on bike and on foot. It's fairly steep and about 1.2 kilometres long. About halfway up, I was in trouble again. Huffing and puffing, I had to stop walking. Eventually, I made it to Pedal's office. Sweating profusely, gasping. They hustle me into an exam office, wipe me down and put the blood pressure cuff on and connect me to the ECG machine. Then Pedals comes in, says, they are going to do a quick ultrasound on me. I said, "I don't know who steepened your hill, but I am definitely not a fan". Pedals laughed, then added he'll be back after the ultrasound. Pedals returned and asked a battery of questions. "I don't like this at all. I am going to set up an angiogram. Before I left the office, Pedals gave me a stern warning – no cycling, no swimming, a slow-paced walk at most. And even your walks should be accompanied. Have your phone with you at all times (which I always do anyhow). It shouldn't take long to get the angiogram. Well, this went well. I wonder what I will learn at the pacemaker clinic.

The pacemaker clinic is down the newly extra steep hill, then up another small hill, so roughly two kilometres total. I went extra slow up the hill and didn't have nearly the struggle with this hill than I did getting to Pedals' office. I told them what happened on the way to Pedals and that he was sending me for an angiogram. They interrogated my pacemaker. It had six alerts on it, meaning that I had six incidents where my heart glitched to some degree. None were correlated with what just happened. I hadn't noticed any of the alerts, either because: I might have been sleeping, they were too brief, or the second pacemaker actually kicked in when it was supposed to. A couple of fun things they do during these interrogations is test the range and responsiveness of the pacemaker. First, they have it zoom up to 150 beats per minute. Those beats I can actually feel because I'm just sitting there. There are no competing body functions like gasping for air, to mask the heart pumping. Too bad that is not an approved exercise protocol. Get your heart rate up to 150 while you just sit there doing nothing. Then they go in the opposite direction, taking the heart rate down to 25 beats. Now that is extra trippy. And you definitely feel those. Buh-BOOM.... buh-BOOM... buh-BOOM... for about 10 seconds. Then it is back to normal. At least on the pacemaker level, everything looked good.

MEET THE WIDOW MAKER

I was initially blanking big time on this entire angiogram adventure beyond that I had three blockages, with two they were really worried about. Then the fog rolled out. I am pretty-sure it was done by Dr. Angio. It's really hard to keep track of all the doctors I've encountered. The nurse noted my chart showed I had a significant weight loss and asked how I managed that. "I practice intermittent fasting," I responded. "Oh, I used to do that. I didn't seem to have any success with it". I said, "That's pretty unusual. Most people just need a few tweaks and then it works great. Regardless, you already look pretty fit and lean, so something is working for you". "What do you mean, tweaks? You are either fasting or you aren't". "Most people just think they should go 16:8 and that's all they need (the 16-hour fasting window and 8 hour eating window). Most people need a shorter eating window or a different fasting protocol. And of course, you need to fast clean". "Different protocols? Fast clean? What are you talking about? None of the videos I watched talk about those things". "I guess today is your lucky day then". I explained the concepts and then a new doctor came in. "Hi, I'm Dr. Special, a resident here in Cardiology. I'm going to be helping with your angiogram". Dr. Special and I had pre-procedure conversation and a moment of confusion that led to a chuckle. She asked how I enjoyed working with a certain doctor and I said very much. In fact, he offered to play some tennis with me when I healed up. Huh? Tennis? I didn't know he played tennis. And he's certainly never invited me. I don't know what to say. Bill seems like a good guy. Bill? Who is Bill? Bill is one of the cardiologists at the other hospital. Who are you talking about? Peter, the Dr. I report to. Two cardiologists, same last name, separate hospitals. We chuckled and moved on.

They did this angiogram through the vein or artery in the wrist. Even though it would prevent me from cycling for a week to 10 days, this was much preferred over the previous method of going through the groin and being walking impaired for a week. Between the antihistamine and sedative, I was my usual chatty, unfiltered self. As much as I wanted to see the Angio screen and watch everything being done, I just couldn't get the proper angle. Dr. Angio finishes and gives Special guidance on how to put the wrist compression device on me. Apparently, they are big on not letting you bleed out like the spurting Knight in Monty Python's Holy Grail movie "It's just a flesh wound!" A couple of nurses walk me back to the room (well, roll me actually) and Dr. Special joins us. Dr. A will be here in a minute to go over your results. After a bit of a wait, Dr. Angio comes in with a printout. I was expecting some high-definition pictures, but this was more like a hand drawn mock-up of the main issues they found. It showed three distinct blockages, none of which were there when I had the angiogram in 2009.

Dr. A explains one is a minor blockage in a minor artery in an awkward spot, so they likely won't even try to fix that. The second it a fairly big blockage in a significant artery, so that needs to be opened. Now the third, explains Dr. Angio., this is called the Widow Maker. It's the most dangerous blockage you can have. I am so confused at this point. All the Intermittent Fasting, change in diet (although still far from perfect) and exercise are supposed to be prophylactic. I ask how this is even possible. Sometimes, it just happens, and we have no explanation. Now, about that Widow Maker blockage. Like many roller-coaster rides or golf course holes, this blockage is called The Widow Maker for a reason. The rides and golf holes are so treacherous in concept that they are apt to leave your wife a widow. However, if this artery in your heart gets fully blocked, there is no conceptual widow created. You are definitely leaving a widow behind. I get to keep the souvenir printout. Thankfully, my Widow Maker blockage was much lower down the artery, so while it was impairing blood flow, I hadn't progressed to full, imminent Widow Maker status yet. To my uneducated eye, all three blockages looked like they were in awkward spots. And it turns out they were. I was going to need stents put in to relieve the blockages. If you aren't familiar with cardiac stents, they use a medically coated wire mesh tube to prop open the artery. And they do the procedure while you are awake.

BREATHE, JUST TRY TO BREATHE

It's Friday, October 12, 2018, and I reported to the hospital for the angioplasty. It is a day procedure. They were going to put two stents in me. As Dr. Angio surmised, the third blockage was deemed too insignificant to address. To do the procedure, they have to use a contrast dye to help them see what is going on with the big board. I have a history of allergic reactions to contrast dyes, so they are supposed to infuse me with a dose of an antihistamine (Do I have to say it? Product placements are still available). The doctor comes in to chat and go through my meds. I was confident in this doc as Dr. Pedals told me this is the doc who works on Pedal's own father. Given Pedals can choose any angioplasty doctor in the city, to me that is a good sign. Doc tells me he guesstimates he has done 20,000 of these procedures, so we'll just call him Dr. 20K. We are going through the meds list and 20k says "Where is your blood thinner?" "I said, I am on the aspirin". No, he says, you need to be on an actual, separate blood thinner. You should have been on this for the entire week before we do the procedure. I respond, "Ummmm, either no one told me, or I just had a major brain fart. I don't remember getting a prescription or the Pharmacy sending me a text that I had a prescription to pick up". And here is when my Spidey sense started tingling and I just knew something was once again going to turn in to another adventure.

The team comes in to prep me for the procedure. You get shaved all over and wiped down with antiseptic, you know, just in case. The woman who shaved me and wiped me down was the same one who shaved and wiped me down prior to the pacemaker surgery five months previous. There were 2 nurses – one was the second shift nurse from the previous surgery (Anastasia, in case you forgot) and the second nurse was new – I'll call her Giggles. Anastasia didn't recognize me at first, so I reminded her of our adventure together, crazy storm, the power outage, the transport ambulance being 6-8 hours late. Then she started remembering, looked at me with her head kind of tilted. Now, I am in no way inferring Anastasia is any type of dog, just trying to present the image of her expressions as we tried to reconnect. Ever see a puppy get confused, and it slowly tilts its head. Then you can see something in its face that seems to say "What the hell? I don't understand what is going on here at all". That was what Anastasia looked like to me. Even Giggles picked up on it and asked what's wrong? Anastasia said she wasn't sure, and she couldn't put her finger on it. Then I said "Oh, I know what it is. I'm much smaller and healthier than when you saw me after surgery. I've lost about 40 pounds but because I also lost a lot of inflammation, it looks like I lost more than that". Then it clicked with her, and the conversation shifted to Anastasia asking not so much about the weight loss (she had zero fat on her) but why this made me disproportionately healthier. And if I was so much healthier, why was she prepping me for a stent procedure? Well, the rest of me was much healthier. My cardiac issues, well, those are another story. Questions and more questions.

MEET GIN STEPHENS, QUEEN OF INTERMITTENT FASTING

Intermittent fasting has become an integral part of my life and recovery. The cardiologist who turned Dr. Pedals on to it told me "Intermittent fasting is the most powerful non-medical medical intervention tool we have". I began to explain the principles of Intermittent Fasting to the nurses. Giggles was interested in the weight loss aspect, and I told them to read two books. Yes, the first was *The Obesity Code* (TOC). The second was a book I had just ordered but hadn't read yet, *Delay, Don't Deny* (DDD) by Gin Stephens. Gin is one of the few people in the book whose name is actually her name. A few of my friends read DDD and raved about it. Gin started and runs a Facebook group based on supporting the book. Just look up the DDD Book Support Group or as of March 2021, her new independent site, www.GinStephens.com/ community. She also lives the IF lifestyle, having lost 80 plus pounds herself. Plus, she's kept it off for five years and counting. I found out about Gin though my work wife, Aly. I had been in one of Dr. Fung's groups, but that didn't end well. Social media. It's kind of hit or miss, right? Work wife had me join the DDD group in March 2018. Of course, the group was much smaller 2+ years ago. Only 31,000 members. I loved the way this group worked. The moderators were amazing. I spent a lot of time learning more about IF, answering questions from other members, and adding my unique sense of humour to the group (which admittedly, not all members get or appreciate). It was an incredibly positive experience and still is. In fact, I became a moderator in the group in January 2020 – the group had just passed 180,000 members. As I write this (August 2022), Gin's written two other books. In the main FB DDD group, there are now over 335,000 members. Why has it grown so fast? Well, Gin is a force of nature. And two, her new book *Fast Feast Repeat* (FFR) is a NY Times best seller. So that helps attract people. If you only buy one book about Intermittent Fasting, buy *FAST, FEAST, REPEAT*. Unless it is a choice between buying this book and Gin's book. Then, of course, buy this one. And a few copies for friends. Oh, wait, you already bought this book. Heck, blow your budget and buy a few copies of each book for those you love.

THE ALLERGY ASPHYXIATION – CLUSTERFUCK 4.0

So back to the prep. I was fully shaved and cleaned. One nurse brought me a larger than normal dose of blood thinners to try to somewhat make up for the fact I should have been taking it all week. A porter comes and wheels me to the operating lab. Ah, the familiar super cold air of the lab so the machines don't overheat. The person I thought was doing my procedure, Dr. 20K, comes in and says, "Meet Dr. Resident. I am training him and he's going to be doing your procedure, OK?" Ummm, again, shouldn't this have been something you discussed with me long before the procedure? It's not like I really have any say in the matter. And so far, my record with residents haven't been great. Well, except Dr. Special, who helped with my angiogram a couple of weeks previous. Yes, I might have developed a slight crush on her. Smart, excellent communication skills. Unfortunately, Dr. Special wasn't scheduled to take part in the angioplasty.

Back to this new resident. He didn't look overly confident to me. You want me to let this guy operate on my heart? I bite my lip. Everyone comes in and running through a variety of checklists. Then they get to "antihistamine administered". Someone shouts out confirmed. I shout out, NOT CONFIRMED! The resident says, "Don't interrupt!" Now I really don't want this guy touching me. I say "Excuse me? I'm certainly interrupting. You're making a mistake that can severely affect me. They gave me a dose of blood thinners. No one gave me an antihistamine; your records are wrong. You aren't doing anything to me until this gets rectified". Doctor 20K steps in. He directs one nurse to go find Anastasia or go to the pharmacy and check what was going on. Maybe 10 minutes later, she comes back (They could have simply phoned) and says "The pharmacy did not dispense any antihistamine. It's been ordered and will be here in a minute". The resident just glared at me. Not a good sign. In my humble opinion, the senior doctor should have booted him at that point and done the procedure himself. Booting the resident may have saved me a lot of grief down the road. Yes, this is more foreshadowing. But I guess we'll never know.

The antihistamine finally arrives. They also give me some mild sedative and finally administer the contrast dye. They re-sterilize my arm, at the catheter insertion point. All of this is done though a vein or artery in my wrist. They manoeuvre little instruments on the end of the catheter through the venous system until it gets to the appropriate places in the heart. Yes, they are wiggling tools around in your heart while you are awake and talking. The general plan is that they get to the blockage, inflate a balloon to create space, then insert the stent. Dr. 20K told me I was getting the latest generation stents called drug-eluting stents. These are stents with an inner coating of a medication. This prevents future clogging of whatever blocks your arteries. They've been around for about a decade, but they keep playing with the coating to make them more effective. I'm guessing this is about the fifth generation of stent. Soon after the procedure starts, Dr. Special comes in to observe. Or at least I think it is her. I generally have a hard enough time figuring out who is who. Never mind with all these masks on and being drugged up. With Covid, having everyone masked up has been very difficult for me recognition-wise. Assuming it was Dr. Special, I guess she got special dispensation from someone. The procedure continues. The combination of sedative and nerves and my natural curiosity about knowing what they are doing pretty much turns off my filters and makes me a little too chatty. I think this further annoys the Resident and amuses the alleged Dr. Special. The Resident seems to have trouble getting the stents where they need to go. I think he is getting some combination of stressed and frustrated.

I'm thinking there should be more input from the Dr. 20K but nope. He essentially had become just an observer. The procedure ends. The Resident basically bolts out of the lab, and I get wheeled back to the recovery room. I have no recollection of either the Resident or 20K checking in on me. That doesn't mean they didn't. They may have. Anastasia's shift either ended or she was dealing with another patient. Only Giggles is around. The standard operating procedure is to monitor the patient for a few hours, make sure they don't spring any leaks, and then release them to the wilds. It didn't take long for me to notice something wasn't right. I tell Giggles I am having trouble breathing. She says, "Your oxygen saturation numbers are great. You are obviously breathing". No, something is definitely wrong. No, you are fine. On Giggles' next check, we go through the same schtik. Same result. She checks the packing and pressure device on my wrist, thanks me for the information about Intermittent Fasting, and sends me off to the mean streets of Toronto.

By the time I get home, I am really struggling with my breathing. I'm just too exhausted to do anything about it. And it is the Sabbath. I basically sleep through Saturday and wake up Sunday. My breathing symptoms haven't eased. Tuesday rolls around and it is time for my regular appointment with Dr. Plié. My post procedure follow-up with Dr. Coif is on Wednesday. Dr Plie agreed that something was off, but I seem to be getting around, so it was more something uncomfortable than urgent. Still, I should go to emergency because I should not have any symptoms. Because almost no one has complications from an angioplasty. Into the ride share I go, off to emergency. While I am waiting to be triaged, this kid takes the seat beside me. If I looked bad, this kid was looking worse than me by a huge margin.

The kid was 15/16 years old. He was trying really hard to drink a large cup of contrast dye for his upcoming CT scan. Me, being me, asked the kid (I'll call him Stiches) what he was in for. Without batting an eye, he says, "Oh, I'm the kid who got stabbed seven times a few weeks ago. You probably heard about me on the news". Nope. Totally missed that one. Had no idea what he was talking about, so I look over at his mom. Is he messing with me? That is usually what I do with people. Mom says nope, 100% truth. Holy crap! Stiches tells me he was going home from getting a haircut and got mugged (Gore warning), then gives me all the details about how the attackers went after him with machetes! One strike went right through his body (he is fairly skinny), he lost about 1/2 his liver, damaged his pancreas, spleen, gall bladder and lost a kidney. It was just a fluke that a couple were walking their dog and came across him bleeding out in the alley. Stiches bled so much that by the time the EMTs got him to the hospital, he had almost no blood left. Now one of his drainage tubes was coming out, so he needs some scans done. The kid was in obvious pain but was so polite and cool as a cucumber. Then he said "I'll be fine. I'm just going to have all these scars". I said don't worry, the chicks will dig them.

We are waiting and waiting. I said to Mom, "I don't want to overstep but I know of something that might help with scar reduction and healing over time". Mom and Grandma said fire away. I started telling them about IF, DDD, Dr. Fung. They started asking all sorts of questions. When I started explaining about how IF makes you generate more growth hormone and how autophagy (a cellular process that is basically the recycle and repurpose function for proteins in the body, unclogging cells and reducing inflammation) does all this healing, they really got interested.

We were in theatre rows - we were in the last row, against the wall, with two more rows in front of us. Maybe 10 people per row. As we are talking, Grandma is taking notes on her smart phone, which I thought was pretty impressive. Both Mom and Grandma express that this sounds other worldly. How can any of this be possible? Then, in a surreal moment, I notice people in front of us are turning around and listening to the conversation. Some time later, this Indian gentleman (IF is truly going worldwide) sitting in front of us says "Dr. Fung is a Rockstar, I've read his books. He's helped many members of my family. You should get the books". We chat some more. This other front-row lady who was also listening gets brave enough to chime in. (Shameless self promotion/pat on the back for her here) "I'm an EMT and everything this gentleman (me) said is true and 100% backed by science. He really knows his stuff". Blush. I only know my stuff because Gin Stephens taught me her stuff. She adds she has been Intermittent Fasting for a year, then went Keto and has dropped 75 lbs. She tells Mom that she now runs her own keto group on FB. I'm positive I am the only one who knows what a Keto group is, but no matter. She comes over to Grandma and helps her order both Gin's books and Fung's books on the spot. I'd plug the EMT's group, but she never said what it is. In a cute moment a bit later, Grandma whispered to me, "Yeah, the books are primarily for him, but to be honest, I could stand to lose a few pounds too". He finally finishes his CT cocktail and gets called in for his scan. I also get called in to whatever awaits me in Emerg. I wish him luck and good health.

Emergency is jam packed. I explain what's going on and they find me a gurney. Eventually, I get into a screening "room" with an actual bed. Or as real a bed as you can get in an emergency room. It's definitely better than a basic gurney. I guess it is more of a bay with a big curtain than a room. I don't know how long I've been in there. It's seeming unlikely I am going to be seen by a doctor anytime soon. Even though I am still struggling with my breathing, I need to get up and do something. I start walking down the hall. So many people look like they could use my bed more than me. Or the little bit of privacy the curtains provide. I'm in my own little world when I hear a woman's voice – Well, hello again! It's Stiches' Mom. They want to keep him overnight to get his tube fixed up. Papa Stiches also arrived. Mom introduces us and we chat a bit. I offer them my room, but they decline. Even if they had accepted, I learned that hospitals kind of frown on patients swapping rooms on their own. Can't imagine why.

The usual tag team of doctors come to see me. Ultimately, they decide to call Cardiology for a consultation. It turns out Dr. Special is on call. "Well, this isn't a good sign. What's going on?" I give her the Cliffs notes version. She orders blood work on me, sends me for a chest x-ray and does an ultrasound on me herself. Everything seems ok, but it obviously isn't. She consults with a senior cardiologist, who doesn't have an opinion on what's causing this. Special gives me a shot of nitroglycerin (aka nitro) to see if that helps. The nitro provides considerable relief. Which is odd because they put in the stents to alleviate my needing drugs like Nitro. I shouldn't need it. Yet I do need it. That should have been a major clue to the senior cardiologist. It seems I am doing better, so they release me. Back into the ride share and home I go, feeling better, but not great.

I manage to get a few hours sleep. Just before noon Wednesday, it's time to head to Dr. Coif's. Back into the ride share I go. Normally to get to Coif or Plié, I do a combination of cycling and subway. It's just not possible at this point. One, I can't breathe, and two, I can't use my wrist where they did the insertion of the surgical tools. Whatever relief I had from the Nitro has long passed. I arrive on time. Reception messages Coif that I don't look good at all. He was caught up with another patient. He told reception to have the Nurse Practitioner check me and he'd join us as soon as possible. For those of you not familiar with Nurse Practitioners, here is the description from the Canadian Nurses

Association website: Nurse practitioners (NPs) are registered nurses who have additional education and nursing experience, which enables them to:

Autonomously diagnose and treat illnesses

Order and interpret tests

Prescribe medications

Perform medical procedures

Now you are up to speed. It was great that I could be seen immediately. What wasn't great is exactly what happens when you get passed between various doctors at the hospital. You have to go through all your medical history again. I go through my history. I suspect she's never had a patient with my colourful history. After hearing me out and checking my vitals, she says, "I need to get Dr. Coif. You are beyond anything I've ever seen". Dr. Coif comes in, looks at me, does a double take (always a comforting move), asks me a couple of questions, and tells me he's calling 911.

The EMTs were literally around the block and arrived quickly. Then Dr. Coif had to convince their supervisor that the prudent move is to let them take me out of zone to the hospital that performed the procedure for me a few days previous. Even though I could walk, the EMTs make you do the gurney run, through the office, down the hallway, into the elevator, down to the ground floor, elevator doors open and of course three people rush in, smashing into me, not looking to see if anyone needs to come out. We finally make it out to the street, into the ambulance. The EMTs and I chat a bit, then I fall asleep. Or at least I hope I was only sleeping. Arriving at the hospital, I go for another gurney ride. The poor EMTs register me, then have to wait until I get admitted to the ER. And wait. And wait. The triage nurse says, "Weren't you here yesterday?" "Sadly, yes". I reply. "Unfortunately, what brought me in yesterday is still going on. I hope we have a better outcome today". One of the transport crew wheels me into a room. They hook up the monitors and it's my turn to wait. And wait. And wait. Eventually, a doctor and an intern come in. The doctor introduces himself as a Head of Something or other. We go through every detail again and he says to me, "Are you sure you are having these symptoms?" Slightly miffed, I respond, "Yep, I'm pretty sure that I am not here for the social aspect. Unless you are holding a rave that I don't know about". The doctors go outside to huddle.

A few minutes later, they return and announce, "We're going to bring in Dr. Echo to give you a thorough ultrasound". Ok, back to the waiting game. Finally, Dr. Echo arrives with the machine and gets to work. The two original doctors watch his every move. After maybe 30 minutes, we have a decision. "Aside from your ribs being abnormally close together, and making this reading more difficult, I don't see anything out of the ordinary". Odd. I've had dozens of ultrasounds for several cardiologists. None of the techs or doctors mentioned anything about my ribs. Whatever. We are back in the "if the doctor can't see it on a test, it must not be happening" mode. The important thing is they still don't know anything that will help me. Head doctor finally says to me "Are you sure you aren't just having an anxiety attack?" Seriously? Yeah, my long-time psychiatrist and family doctor couldn't recognize an anxiety attack. Basically, they were saying I was making this all up. Question. If the Nitro was helpful to me yesterday, why not give it to me again while you try to figure this out? I mean, wouldn't the fact that the Nitro did something mean it wasn't anxiety? Or just something I made up? Because, shocker, all they would do is keep checking the same things over and over. Oh, that cognitive bias. It's everywhere. They discharge me and I'm fuming.

You might wonder where my cardiologist was in all this? Good question. Pedals was on a speaking tour in Asia. Head of Something or other doctor apparently eventually messaged him to see if he had any ideas. (Finally, some outside the box thinking). Thursday morning, Dr. Pedals' assistant calls me and says, "Stop taking the blood thinner immediately and take some antihistamines. Dr. Pedals will call you in a couple of hours after his talk". Well ok. About two hours after taking the antihistamine, my symptoms start to ease. Dr. Pedals finally calls "I'm sorry you had to go through all this. It's a real no brainer. You were having an allergic reaction to the blood thinner medication. The antihistamine they gave you for the contrast dye masked it and by the time you were out of the procedure, it was wearing off. It's a well-known side effect of that drug" I thanked him and asked, "If it is well-known, why didn't they know what was going on? He tried to tell me I was simply having an anxiety attack" Dr. Pedals was less than pleased to hear this. "It's a big miss for sure. Stay off the thinners. I'll be back Monday, and I'll huddle with a couple of my colleagues to get a better drug choice for you. And don't be afraid to take the antihistamines. It takes a while for the drug to clear your system".

Friday morning, Dr. Pedals' assistant calls again, "Come in Tuesday morning, be prepared to stay a few hours because we have to squeeze you in". Tuesday rolls around and I am feeling so much better that I no longer need the antihistamine. Dr. Pedals comes in and we catch up. He talks about his conferences a bit and jokes about how his roaming/messaging charges are going to be through the roof because of me. I tell him I am not even on the antihistamine anymore, which turns out to be a good thing. We are going to try a new medication. If I were still on the antihistamine, we wouldn't know if I was reacting to it. He wrote me a new prescription. Then he gave me the added instructions I would likely know in a few hours if I was having a reaction to it, so keep the antihistamines close. If this doesn't work, we'll find something else. Thankfully, I had no reaction. These eluting stents are supposed to keep the pipes open and flowing for years. Add in all the health and weight loss benefits from Intermittent Fasting, plus exercising my body and brain, it should be smooth sailing from here on in, right? Right? I said RIGHT?

After all this, nothing else could possibly happen to me. Yeah, sure. Keep telling yourself this. But wait! I know I am into a bit of foreshadowing, but what's with the gloom and doom? I forgot to add my faith to my smooth sailing formula. What about my faith? My trust in God? That if I have "bitachon" (the Hebrew word for faith as opposed to bitcoin), all is for the good, even if it doesn't look like it. Some people just have a natural orientation to this mindset. Others, like me and my buddy Mr. Privacy, really have to grind at it even though we both strongly believe in God. Yes, coming back to life repeatedly is a huge victory/reward. But having things work out in other aspects of life such as income and relationships, are also required for a quality of life. Will that happen to me?

MR. AND MRS. CALCUTTA CHIME IN AGAIN

The Calcuttas offered this frame of reference. "The Hebrew word for 'life' is 'chaim'. When one Jew toasts another, we say 'l'chaim' - to life. Within the word chaim is contained one of G-d's holy name. And that G-d's name is at the heart of 'life' is surely significant. If one always remembers that G-d (or whatever force you believe in) is at the core of his or her life, no matter what may happen, he or she will surely succeed. Because, no matter what problem may arise, he or she is never alone. The Almighty is always with you - to guide and protect you! May G-d bless you with good health and happiness and with peace and prosperity. May we always share in only joyous occasions." I have my team of angels that have gotten me this far. The question is, are they going to keep me status quo or help me move forward? What do you think?

THE BRAIN TRAINERS

Before I leave, I want to give you some added background on my adventures with the Brain Trainers, then some of the benefits of intermittent fasting. I called Dr. Narrow and his associates the Brain Trainers, as this is what they did for me. Tried to retrain my brain. But first they had to assess me to get a clearer picture. I don't recall the majority of the specific tests but almost all of it was some sort of comparative functional testing. Even back then, science had a pretty-good idea of what functions are processed in what parts of the brain. They have decades of this kind of data so you can standardize it and see where the person fits against expected norms. A psychologist developed a program to test your right brain against the left, right ear versus left, right hand versus left, etc. One of the first tests was just simple finger tapping on a counting device. How many times can you tap in a minute? First with a dominant hand finger and then repeat with the non-dominant hand finger. I think they did three fingers on each hand. I don't know the number parameters but to illustrate the point, say you are right hand dominant. A person within "normal" parameters could be expected to be able to do 100 taps with an index finger per minute, plus or minus. The expected number for the non-dominant index finger would be dominant hand minus 30%, or roughly 70 taps per minute. My dominant hand score was like 50 – worse than the expected for a non-dominant hand.

My left hand was even worse. Ok, we were beginning to understand I had a fine motor skill issue. Among other issues. Thus began my new reality that something was actually not working with my body. I wasn't lazy!!! The working theory was that I had a stroke just before or just after I was born. And no one noticed. That's a pretty big miss.

This really was pretty mind blowing. It took me about six months before I was able to bring myself to sit down with Dr. Narrow and discuss what might happen next. It was going to be a long road. The program essentially was a progressive and cumulative series of tasks that forced me to use the damaged parts of my brain and encourage them to work. The goal is to rewire your brain. Today we call this encouraging neuroplasticity. Some of these exercises were just plain awful. More than once, the task was so difficult that I either almost passed out or vomited. It was pretty exhausting. There was not one session where I went home and could not do anything other than just crash.

I endured about three or four years of working with the learning specialists (at a cost of about $40,000, mostly out of my pocket). It got me to a point where I earned a geography degree (no small feat being colour blind), a certification in Adult Ed and an MBA with a double major in Marketing and Finance. After I graduated with my undergrad degree, I ran into my one of my high school English teachers (Mrs. Mean). I told her what I had been diagnosed with and finally earned a degree. Instead of congratulating me, she just kind of sneered at me like "Learning disabled? What a load of crap. You're just lazy". Once some people get an idea in their head, it's never leaving. Cognitive rigidity fever is everywhere. Regardless of how much I recover, my brain will never be where it is supposed to be. Although I have to say at this point, I seem to be pretty fortunate with where my brain is at. Because this is a Fred kind of story, there is a parallel story to the Brain Trainers, revolving mostly around the associate I primarily worked with. You will read more about this in the chapters Dr. Scam, World Class Shyster, and after that, Dr. Scam on The Lam.

I always got along with Dr. Narrow. He was first rate. He also had a couple of underlings. At least one of them was a PhD student he was advising. Now for as much benefit as I derived working with the Brain Trainers, I feel I left...or rather THEY left a lot on the table. My primary contact (the Ph.D. student) would no longer return my calls, or the admin assistant said he was now too busy to work with me. Sadly, my adventures in Brain Training just petered out. It left a bitter taste in my mouth but there was nothing I could do except try to use what I'd learned. Of course, I had no idea how much was left on the table until a couple of years after I moved to Toronto. And now that I am today years old, the tastes are even more bitter. I am continuously finding ways to rinse out the bad taste and plow forward.

DR. SCAM, WORLD CLASS SHYSTER

The Dr. Scam, as I not-so-fondly call him now, told me he had a masters or PhD already from another university and had decided to switch fields from whatever he was studying (maybe divinity or theology) to psychology. I thought he was a very smart but quirky guy. But just how quirky was ultimately a shocker. Dr. Scam always brought two or three beautiful dogs to our sessions. He told me they were his & that they were prize winning show dogs. Dr. Scam often invited me to the shows but to be honest, I had no real interest in attending. I'm actually quite allergic to dogs. And cats. And nuts. It is quite a list. Finally, I figured if I just went to one, he'd stop asking me. We made plans to meet up. Which turned out to be easier said than done. I couldn't find him. Ultimately, I ran into one of my MBA buddies, who as it turns out, was into show dogs and owned some prize winners himself. He knows everyone on the circuit. He asked what brought me to the show and I told him my buddy was showing his dogs. We quickly figured out he knew my guy. He told me my guy was a glorified dog sitter. Someone else owned the dogs! While it seemed weird, it didn't set off a big red flag for me. I gave people too much benefit of the doubt. When I went to my next session, he swore up and down he was there. I didn't mention my classmate had outed him. It had no impact on anything I was doing and if the guy had a fantasy about owning show dogs, I wasn't going to burst his bubble.

However, Dr. Scam kept trying to involve me in non-brain training activities. He shared with me that he had invested in a Christmas tree farm with another guy. Would I like to come out with him and work on raising the barn with him? Another project I had no interest in, so I made it clear in no uncertain words that this was a no go. He always seemed to have these outside projects going on and I wondered how he had time to do his course work, see patients and operate a farm among other things. This adventure sort of faded into the background. Until it showed up again.

Dr. Scam's next undertaking was talking to me about making money. I mean, I was a financial planner at the time so it kind of made sense. Eventually, he moved the conversations to non-traditional investing (now better known as multi-level marketing or MLM). After a few weeks, he said something along the line of "I have a buddy who has done some really interesting investing and is giving a talk about it next week. Would you like to go?" I thought it was a good idea to keep current. And it was. It turned out to be a good idea to keep an eye on the latest multi-level marketing game my clients might get exposed to. It took a while to fully expose itself as a scam and once it did, I left the meeting. For an initial investment of $3600, you can get an inventory of gold jewelry to resell and ask other people to pony up $3600 so they can do the same. UGH. Didn't see Dr. Scam for a few weeks after but when I did, I gave him an earful. It was shortly after that the calls stopped being returned & appointments went unbooked or he no showed. I should have had a sit down with Dr. Narrow at that point. Not sure why I didn't. I guess I was kinda burned out from all the brain training, going back to university and a breakup - you know, normal life stuff – that I didn't have anything left in the tank to deal with this. Today, (in 2020) I could deal with it. Because I have intermittent fasting as my superpower. And I will happily and enthusiastically share my superpower with anyone. Except, of course, the super villains.

DR. SCAM ON THE LAM

A couple of years after I moved to Toronto, I get a call from Dr. Narrow. He was calling about my outstanding bill, about $5,000. Huh? Ten years and you are calling now? Besides, I had paid everything through a special bursary I got for my learning disabilities. To the best of my knowledge, Dr. Scam billed the foundation directly. Unless he hadn't. Or more accurately, he had billed the foundation, but nothing went to the clinic. "Dammit!" cried Dr. Narrow. "Not you too!" It seemed Dr. Scam had somehow been cooking the books. He was apparently direct billing to his own account, not the clinic's account. I had no idea. And according to Dr. Narrow, he had done this a lot. And by a lot it seems he had done this to well over a dozen patients. Not sure how it went unnoticed. I felt bad for Dr. Narrow. At least he had the resources to go after Dr. Scam.

About a year after that, my mom calls and says there is a guy at the house trying to get in touch with me to talk to me about Dr. Scam. How he found my mom or me is pretty disturbing. What happened to doctor-patient confidentiality? At this point I hadn't seen Scam in well over 10 years, so I wasn't current on him anyhow. Regardless, I told mom to give him my number. That conversation would lead to a slight nickname change. Soon I found myself talking to an incredibly despondent man. He had gone into a business venture with Dr. Scam, who had also cooked his books and disappeared. What business, you ask? This was the poor guy who went into the Christmas tree farm with Dr. Scam. Dr. Scam often talked about how successful it was and how proud he was to have raised a barn. Dr. Scam took this guy for everything he had. According to the farmer, Scam had somehow forged a bunch of documents as to who owned the property and eventually froze the guy out, but not before borrowing the maximum he could against the business and property. The Christmas tree guy said knew five other people who had also been bilked out of significant amounts of cash. He told me there was a Canada-wide arrest warrant out for the newly renamed Dr. Scam on the Lam. I felt bad for everyone he had scammed and sad that I had nothing I could offer him. Occasionally I'll do an online search using Dr. Scam's legal name, but it is a fairly common name and I never find anything of substance. Or at least what I think is his legal name. Hopefully, Karma catches up with him and makes things right with those he screwed over. Oh, and if you see Dr. Scam in your travels, please let me know.

YES, I FULLY UNDERSTAND PAIN

Upon reflection, I understand that all the following may have seemed like really negative events. Ok, they were negative events. But I was only viewing them in the time frame of said events. Now that I can look at them in hindsight, I'm trying to reframe these as positive events – mindset is your greatest superpower. Now, I see these negative events were all preparing me in some form or other for *The Summer I Died Twenty Times*. And its aftermath. Or is it aftermaths? I'm not sure. The point is, it's really important to put into context how unbelievably awful this dying stuff is. I haven't exactly had a trauma-free life. But now I see all these traumas as having had a purpose. In fact, I've flirted with death a number of times, so it provides some context. These are some of the traumas I've experienced, each pretty awful in their own right. And each somehow was a contributor to my current set of superpowers. Here goes:

I've been T-boned in a car at 40 mph. I've been on the bottom of a pile in Rugby (called a ruck) with some very-large angry men giving me the stomps multiple times (and no, I didn't deserve it). One of my teammates took a cheap shot at one of the opposing players and they thought I did. I would NEVER! I've taken an elbow to the face that broke my orbital bone. Also in rugby, I've had a guy cheap shot me with a knee to the ribs that broke 4 of them. I had a buddy who played NHL hockey accidently hit me with a slap shot that shattered my shin pad and left me with a horrible bone bruise. Now a bone bruise doesn't sound so bad but let me tell you, holy fuck it hurts. I think this happened to NFL superstar Rob Gronkowski the other year and Rob is a tough tough guy. And Rob went down like he was shot and missed a few games. The point is that it is unbelievably painful because some things just hurt disproportionately more than they seem they should. Like stepping on Lego in the dark or stubbing a toe.

DEATH BY CAT WITH A BONUS CONCUSSION

While cycling, I've been hit by a car multiple times, as well as a truck, and a cat. Not all at the same time, of course. And yes, a freaking cat. The truck and the cat were the worst. I was even taken out by a gust of wind that propelled me down a hill at 40 plus mph, with my narrowly missing getting garrotted by a hydro pole guide wire. I wasn't able to avoid the accompanying severe case of road rash, which led to me getting my second Covid shot while dripping blood all over the pharmacy.

The truck was the first time I truly thought I was dead. I saw it at the last second and tried to escape by jumping over my handlebars. I didn't make it. The truck slammed into me. I spun in the air a few times like a helicopter blade. I slammed to the ground and skidded on the pavement until I crashed headfirst into a curb, which stopped me pretty abruptly. My helmet split in half. I remember thinking, "Am I dead?" Then I concluded no, because being dead couldn't possibly hurt this much. Little did I know. At least the driver got out to help me. It was pretty obvious he'd been drinking. Since I moved to Toronto, I've subsequently been hit or bumped off my bike a few more times. Except here, the drivers just bolted. Life in the big city I guess.

The cat hitting me is far and away the most ridiculous story but without a doubt the most painful. I was cycling home from work around 10 PM. I used to challenge myself to beat my previous times (yeah, I wanted to be the next Lance Armstrong, except steroid free). I was chugging along when I saw a big tomcat walking to the edge of the centre boulevard. I slowed a bit and flashed my helmet light at it. The cat stopped and sat down, so I got back up on my pedals and resumed trying to set a new world record. Just as I got near his position, the stupid fucker bolted and went right under my front wheel. I believe the phrase is flipping me ass over tea kettle. I slammed down on my back and head and skidded down the street, still tangled in my bike.

I don't know how long I was out. I do remember coming to and seeing a line-up of cars behind me with no one getting out to help me. In their defense, it was a bit of a sketchy neighbourhood but still. Actually, there is no defense. They were just a bunch of douchebags. Finally, some stoner came running over from across the centre boulevard and helped me untangle from the bike. (Insert total stoner voice here) "Are you ok Dude? That was fucking spectacular! You totally flipped in the air". He helped me to the curb and left me. I guess he had the munchies or something. Everything hurt, even my fingernails. Amazingly, except for severe road rash, nothing was broken. But obviously I added another concussion to the ledger. Oh, except for my bike. It was trashed. I hope that was the last of that stupid cat's nine lives.

There was also this medical adventure. I woke up during an eye surgery because the anesthetist screwed up royally. Did I mention I am a redhead aka a gingy? It is well documented that redheads need more gas to keep us under along with more numbing to stop us feeling pain. I think at the dentist, I need 2x the normal dose to freeze me. It's not a new concept, dumbass anesthetist. I couldn't signal the docs who kept cutting my eye muscle. I cannot describe how much that hurt. Have you ever watched a football game and the players go out of bounds into a camera, but the producer doesn't change cameras fast enough & the world turns upside down until they switch cameras?

That is what happened to me because they were moving my eye as they cut the surrounding muscle until I figured out to start slamming my hand. A nurse said, "OMG, is he awake? The doc stopped cutting and asked, "Are you awake?" I game him a thumbs up and he screamed "FUCK, Gas now!" Now that was insane pain and yet nothing compared to these undying experiences. By the way, there was no way to hold these "professionals" accountable for their gross negligence, a theme that would be repeated during this continually dying adventure. In the US, I could have sued their asses off. Mental note 1: Have all future surgeries in the US. Mental note 2: I mentioned these experiences to reinforce that I have a truly world class grasp of pain and general awfulness. All those experiences combined, and multiplied hundreds of times just can't accurately describe how awful it was literally coming back from the dead.

THE SECRET WORLD OF NON-SCALE VICTORIES (NSVS)

Now, on to the best parts of intermittent fasting. As Gin often says "IF is the health plan with a side benefit of weight loss". Every day in the Delay Don't Deny fasting group, we run a variety of threads. Everything from Success Stories to Ask a Moderator (the thread I often moderate) to Mindset Matters to the Non-Scale Victories (NSVs) thread. NSVs are victories people notice beyond the scale being the only point of progress reference. Using NSVs is leveraging your mindset superpower to its maximum potential. A typical NSV thread day involved 100 plus submissions! Day after Day, week after week, month after month, people share their benefits from choosing the Intermittent fasting lifestyle.

I have my own exhaustive list of NSVs which I am sharing below. I will likely miss a few but these are real, and thousands of others have experienced similar NSVs, so I am not an exception to the rule. Note: Not everyone experiences all of these, nor do they get them to the same degree. Your mileage may vary:

- Resting pulse went from mid 90s to mid 60s
- BP down to 95/60
- Hair is softer
- Hair colour going back to its original orange
- Dry eyes & crusty stuff abated
- My eyes look clearer

- Day and night vision is better (except oddly for glare – it's worse)
- All body aches cleared (and given the inflammation from this recent surgery, which was brutal, that is saying something)
- Down from size 48 pants to 38 (and dropping)
- Increased energy & mental clarity
- Decreased snot rockets (usually pronounced when exercising)
- Decreased sweating except when exercising – then the floodgates open
- Ha1c went from 6.9 to 5.2
- Brain fog/Writer's block cleared (obviously it has cleared because you are reading this)
- My Type 2 diabetes has reversed itself (aka I am no longer diabetic)
- Diabetic retinopathy healed up
- Asthma has gone
- Sleep apnea is gone (along with snoring and fitful sleeps)
- Skin tags are gone
- Sleeping through the night 4 or 5 times a week
- Arterial plaque is reversing
- Scars are disappearing

This is a list of what others have reported. Over and over again. I don't need some medical study to prove to me that IF is, as Gin Stephens says, the health plan with a side benefit of weight loss.

NSVs Reported by Category

1. Body size/Recomposition
    a. Airplanes seats (no more need for seat extenders or paying for 2 seats, or not being able to use the drop trays because they hit your belly.)
    b. Barber/hair dressing chairs,

    c. Bracelets, necklaces, rings now fit

    d. Fitting into cars, using the seatbelts and getting in/out of cars

    e. Fitting into restaurant booths instead of being forced to use chairs (and being terrified the chairs won't hold you,

    f. Being able to shop off the rack in normal clothing stores and not needing expensive alterations of all types,

    g. Having the energy to do gardening, yard work etc., Plus the strength to get up and down, and even work on your knees.

    h. Vision improving and less reliance on glasses,

    i. Being able to fully hug those you like to hug,

    j. Mobility in general,

    k. Fitting into seats at the movies,

    l. Packing on muscle

    m. Playing with kids/grand kids, getting up and down from the floor, chasing them around,

    n. Not needing special order shoes,

    o. Easily going up and down stairs,

    p. Walk down airplane aisles without crashing into every armrest (one of my personal favourites),

    q. Needing to resize watch bands, bracelets.

2. Bloating/Fluid Retention

    a. Gastrointestinal issues, diagnosed or not, disappear,

    b. No more compression stockings,

    c. No more general swelling or decreased inflammation in general,

    d. No foot/leg swelling after travel (any type where you can't walk around),

    e. Blood pressure decreases,

    f. Heart rate decrease,

    g. Lymphatic problems greatly reducing.

3. Clothes/shopping
    a. Eating/Food
    b. Shopping/meal planning/time spent in kitchen making meals greatly decreased
    c. Good food tastes better, processed food tastes junkier,
    d. Improved portion control,
    e. Appetite correction – your body tells you when you are full/satiated,
    f. Don't obsess about food anymore,
    g. Less guilt with people seeing you eating,
    h. Save $$$$$ (which is great in these hyper inflationary times),
    i. Buy higher quality foods (more natural/raw),
    j. Buy better quality clothes, which go on sale, unlike the oversize clothing that rarely goes on sale.

4. Dental
    a. Gingivitis reversal (and this is big, as studies show gingivitis can lead to cardiac issues),
    b. TMJ resolving itself,
    c. Whiter teeth,
    d. Less plaque making dental cleanings easier and quicker,
    e. Less cavities (who doesn't want less cavities?),
    f. Less tooth sensitivity.

5. Endurance
    a. Energy levels off the charts,
    b. Improved focus/mental clarity,
    c. Increased endurance,

  d. Little to no post workout soreness (Delayed Onset Muscle Soreness or DOMS),

  e. Sex drive and performance, reported by both men and women,

  f. Packing on muscle,

  g. Recover faster and easier from exertions,

  h. Working out fasted becomes the norm.

6. Medical condition reversals or significant improvements

  a. Autoimmune (Rheumatoid arthritis is a huge one),

  b. Adrenal fatigue,

  c. Seasonal allergies,

  d. Bells Palsy,

  e. Brain fog & memory issues,

  f. Chronic fatigue,

  g. Crones, IBS

  h. Cycles normalized,

  i. Type 2 diabetes,

  j. Dry eyes,

  k. ED/Libido (both sides of the aisle kids),

  l. Erratic heart/Arrhythmias,

  m. Excessive sweating,

  n. Fatty liver,

  o. Glaucoma,

  p. High blood pressure,

  q. Body-wide inflammation,

  r. Joint pain,

  s. Foot/leg cramping, cramps in general,

  t. Migraines, headaches, sinus headaches, sinus infections,

  u. Nerve pain, neuropathy,

  v. Night sweats,

  w. No colds/flus,

  x. Osteoarthritis,

y. Osteoporosis,

z. PCOS,

aa. Perimenopause/menopause symptoms decreased,

bb. Plantar fasciitis,

cc. Sciatica, Thyroid normalized,

dd. Uterine fibroids, Varicose/spider veins reduced,

ee. Weak bladder reversals,

7. Medications decreased or no longer required (Remember, always consult with your medical professionals before adjusting your medications)

a. Allergy meds,

b. Anxiety,

c. Blood pressure,

d. Cholesterol,

e. Depression,

f. Estrogen,

g. Eye medications,

h. Heart burn/GERD,

i. Immune suppressants,

j. Insulin,

k. Metformin,

l. Pain relievers,

m. Puffers/asthma meds,

n. Anti-rejection drugs,

o. Steroids,

p. Supplements,

q. Testosterone/Estrogen,

r. Thyroid,

s. Ulcers

8. Mental Health

a. Improved mood/ attitude/ tempers/ patience/ self-esteem/ confidence/ joy

9. Physical changes/body recomposition

a. Belly fat/Back fat,
b. Being able to cross one's legs,
c. Finding that you have a lap,
d. No cracking joints,
e. No restless legs,
f. Reduced fidgeting,
g. Sitting cross legged,

10. Nails
a. Many report their nails were stronger, no longer cracked or tore,
b. One lady reported her nails were now too strong to bite anymore,
c. No more ingrown toenails,
d. No more toe fungus/discoloured toenails.

11. Hair
a. Grows faster,
b. Less body hair (less shaving/waxing),
c. Less gray and/or hair returns to its natural colour,
d. Less hair loss,
e. Hair is stronger/less brittle,

12. Skin - People report that overall, their skin is much improved. Specifics are:
a. Acne
b. Callouses/heal cracking
c. Cellulite
d. Cold sores, heal faster,
e. Dandruff
f. Eczema
g. Jowels, turkey necks
h. Keloids
i. Moles
j. Oily skin
k. Pores shrinking

l. Psoriasis

m. Scar removal

n. Skin tags disappear

o. Softer/smoother

p. Stretch marks/ surgical scars/ caesarian scars vanishing

q. Tightening

r. Warts, blisters

13. Sleep/Rest Recovery

a. Better quality sleep

b. Sleep apnea reversed

c. No more snoring (men & women)

d. No daytime swan or naps required

And of course, I can't forget how IF has ramped up my neuroplasticity. This alone has given me a good chance of getting my life back. I know many of you won't accept this as proof IF works. It's like the doctors who can't give credence to a patient's symptoms unless they can see it on a test. You need some sort of human trials documented in a medical journal. It's just not going to happen. No company is going to fund IF studies because there is no money to be made. There are no IF medications. No supplements. No costly programs. Thus, there is no incentive to fund studies that can't be monetized. Further, as IF gets people healthier, it will likely cut into existing revenue streams as people need less and less medication., I can't emphasize enough how much IF has altered my life so positively. Maybe it can alter your life too.

ABOUT THE AUTHOR

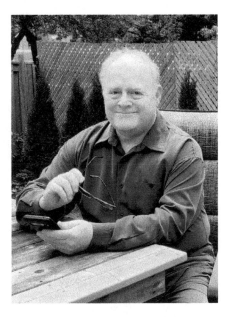

Currently living in Toronto, Ontario, Fred Rutman is a former marketer, consultant and professor (marketing and finance). He is also an avid intermittent faster, which he credits with saving his life. And improving the lives of countless others he works with.

NOTE FROM THE AUTHOR

Word-of-mouth is crucial for any author to succeed. If you enjoyed *The Summer I Died Twenty Times*, please leave a review online—anywhere you are able. Even if it's just a sentence or two. It would make all the difference and would be very much appreciated.

Thanks!
Fred Rutman

We hope you enjoyed reading this title from:

BLACK ❀ ROSE
writing™

www.blackrosewriting.com

Subscribe to our mailing list – *The Rosevine* – and receive **FREE** books, daily deals, and stay current with news about upcoming releases and our hottest authors.
Scan the QR code below to sign up.

Already a subscriber? Please accept a sincere thank you for being a fan of Black Rose Writing authors.

View other Black Rose Writing titles at www.blackrosewriting.com/books and use promo code **PRINT** to receive a **20% discount** when purchasing.